The Clueless Vegetarian

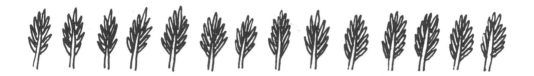

A Cookbook for the Aspiring Vegetarian

EVELYN RAAB

FIREFLY BOOKS

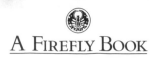

A FIREFLY BOOK

Published by Firefly Books Ltd. 2012

First printing

Publisher Cataloging-in-Publication Data (U.S.)

Raab, Evelyn.
The clueless vegetarian : a cookbook for the aspiring vegetarian / Evelyn Raab.
2nd ed.
[216] p. : ill. ; cm.
Includes index.
Summary: Vegetarian cooking explained with helpful illustrations and step-by-step instruction.
ISBN-13: 978-1-55407-995-7 (pbk.)
1. Vegetarian cooking. 2. Cookbooks. I. Title.
641.5/636 dc23   TX837.R334   2012

Library and Archives Canada Cataloguing in Publication

Raab, Evelyn
The clueless vegetarian : a cookbook for the aspiring
vegetarian / Evelyn Raab. -- 2nd ed.
Includes index.
Previous ed. also published under title: Basic vegetarian cooking.
Toronto : Prospero Books, c2008.
ISBN-13: 978-1-55407-995-7
 1. Vegetarian cooking. 2. Cookbooks. I. Title.
TX837.R318 2012   641.5'636   C2011-906859-1

Published in the United States by
Firefly Books (U.S.) Inc.
P.O. Box 1338, Ellicott Station
Buffalo, New York 14205

Published in Canada by
Firefly Books Ltd.
66 Leek Crescent
Richmond Hill, Ontario L4B 1H1

Illustrations: George A. Walker
Design: Jean Lightfoot Peters

Printed in Canada

The publisher gratefully acknowledges the financial support for our publishing program by the Government of Canada through the Canada Book Fund as administered by the Department of Canadian Heritage.

Contents

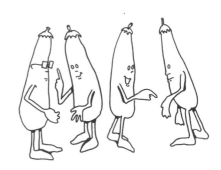

Introduction

So you're a vegetarian. Or you're thinking about it. Or maybe you live with a vegetarian.

But you don't want to eat only weird food. Or spend all day cooking it. Congratulations, you've come to the right place.

The Clueless Vegetarian is designed for vegetarians who love good food cooked from scratch but who also want to have a life. This book is filled with simple recipes for just about everything you might ever want to eat and a few things you wouldn't touch with a 10-foot pole. You'll find recipes for lasagna and chili and burritos. There are curries and casseroles. There are hearty soups and satisfying snacks. There are even some truly decadent desserts.

There are, of course, also recipes for tofu, tempeh and textured vegetable protein (TVP). Because you should know about this stuff. Really.

If you're just switching to a vegetarian diet, *The Clueless Vegetarian* gives you the straightforward nutritional information you need to help you make good food choices — without obsessing over it. There are hints for concocting vegetarian versions of some of your favorite dishes and suggestions for preparing meals for the mixed household. You'll even find survival tips and cooking advice that's just plain useful for anyone, vegetarian or not.

Now let's start with the basics, shall we? We'll save the tempeh for later. It's best to work up to these things gradually.

Icons Used in This Book

The recipe contains dairy ingredients, such as milk, cheese or yogurt.

The recipe contains eggs.

The recipe is vegan, which means that it does not contain eggs, dairy or other animal products or that it *can* be prepared as a vegan dish by omitting animal products or using the suggested substitutions. If a recipe is identified with D, E *and* V it means that a vegan variation of the recipe is suggested.

Quick Fix!, which is a recipe that can be thrown together from scratch in 30 minutes or less.

The recipe is gluten free.

1. Vegetarian Survival Skills

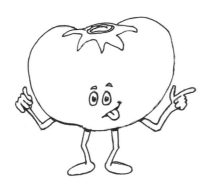

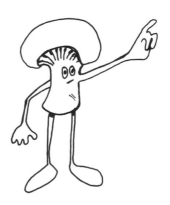

What Kind of Vegetarian Are You, Anyway?

There's more than one way to be a vegetarian. The choice depends, of course, on your deep moral convictions, your sense of spirituality and your cosmic connection to the totality of the universe. It also depends on what you like to eat and what sort of diet you're prepared to follow.

Vegan

Vegans eat vegetables, fruits and grains only. That's it. Nothing that has ever had anything to do with any sort of living creature. No eggs, no dairy, not even honey. Many, but not all, of the recipes in this book are suitable for a vegan diet.

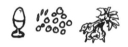

Ovo-Vegetarian

They eat vegetables, fruits, grains and eggs. No dairy.

Lacto-Vegetarian

They eat vegetables, fruits, grains and dairy products. This includes milk, cheese, yogurt and butter. No eggs.

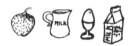

Lacto-Ovo Vegetarian

They eat vegetables, fruits, grains, eggs and dairy products. So, basically anything except actual meat, poultry and fish.

Occasional Vegetarian

They might include chicken and/or fish in their diet (in addition to vegetables, grains, eggs and dairy products) or simply indulge in the occasional burger without feeling too guilty about it.

Living Vegetarianly: Some Helpful Hints

Eat a wide variety of foods. If you are finicky, creeped out by unfamiliar flavors or squeamish about trying new things, now is the time to get over it. While a vegetarian diet doesn't have to be a non-stop exotic adventure, you'll be missing a lot if you don't expand your horizons and take full advantage of all the wonderful vegetarian possibilities out there.

Whenever possible choose whole, unrefined foods. Buy fresh fruits and vegetables in season, natural cheeses and whole-grain breads. The less someone else has fiddled around with your food, the better. This is good advice for anyone, vegetarian or not.

Make your calories count. If you're going to squander extra calories on something, wouldn't you rather it be something absolutely wonderful, like a decadent dessert or some fabulous pasta, rather than a bag of simulated salt and vinegar potato chips?

If you've been invited to someone's home for dinner, tell them beforehand that you are a vegetarian and what, exactly, you will eat. This is no time to be shy. Your host/hostess will appreciate your being straightforward. Really. Even better, offer to bring a vegetarian dish to share, thus guaranteeing that there will be at least one thing you can eat while introducing your friends to something new and delicious.

Teach your friends and family how to make vegetarian versions of familiar foods. Show them how to use tofu or tempeh in a stir-fry instead of meat, let them taste your veggie burrito or invite them to your home for a completely non-weird vegetarian meal. They'll never even miss the meat.

When you're planning a meal, stop thinking meat, potato and two vegetables. Instead, make a dinner out of several side dishes. You can create a meal with soup as the centerpiece and accompany it with some good bread, a salad and a couple of tasty appetizers. Or better yet, do all appetizers. After all, who doesn't love to nibble?

The Vegetarian Food Guide

These basic guidelines, based on Canada's Food Guide, can help you determine whether your diet is on the right track. There is, however, enough flexibility built into it to allow for the little personal idiosyncrasies (maybe you hate yogurt but love lentils) that make us all so wonderfully unique.

The guide below is an outline of the complete dietary requirements for a lacto-ovo vegetarian for a single day. You don't have to fit every single food group into every single meal. Instead, take your eating habits over the course of the whole day, including snacks, into consideration. Does the idea of eight servings of grain products sound outrageous? It's not. Just 1 cup (250 mL) of pasta counts as two servings, and a whole bagel is another two — you're halfway there already.

Grain Products
6 to 8 servings per day

Vegetables and Fruits
7 to 10 servings per day

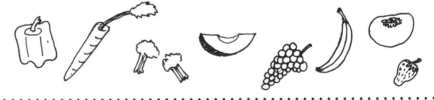

Legumes, Nuts, Seeds, Eggs and Soy
2 to 3 servings per day

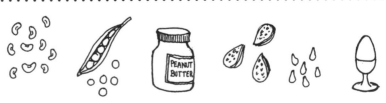

Milk and Alternatives
2 to 3 servings per day

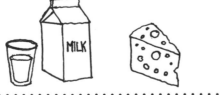

This guide is designed for a healthy, average adult. Children, pregnant or lactating women and teens should consult a doctor or nutritionist for more specific info. And keep in mind that nutritional guidelines are constantly changing; keep up to date with the latest information, both in print and online, if you want to make sure you're eating right.

Grain Products

6 to 8 servings per day (make at least half of these whole grain)
Bread, cereal, rice and pasta
Serving size: 1 slice bread, ½ bagel, pita or tortilla; ½ cup (125 mL) cooked pasta, couscous or rice; 1 oz. (30 g) cold cereal, ¾ cup (175 mL) hot cereal.

Vegetables and Fruits

7 to 10 servings per day
Fresh, frozen or canned vegetables or fruit, or fruit or vegetable juice
Serving size: 1 medium whole fruit (apple, orange, banana), ½ cup (125 mL) chopped raw or cooked vegetables, ½ cup (125 mL) fruit or vegetable juice, 1 cup (250 mL) leafy salad, ¼ cup (60 mL) dried fruit.

Legumes, Nuts, Seeds, Eggs and Soy

2 to 3 servings per day
Legumes (like beans and lentils), nuts, seeds, soy products (like tofu or tempeh), eggs.
Serving size: ¾ cup (175 mL) cooked beans, lentils, tofu or tempeh, 2 eggs, 2 tbsp. peanut butter or nut butters; ¼ cup (60 mL) shelled nuts and seeds.

Milk and Alternatives

2 to 3 servings per day
Milk, yogurt, soft cheeses (like ricotta or cottage cheese), hard cheeses (like cheddar or Swiss)
1 cup (250 mL) milk or fortified soy beverage; ¾ cup (175 mL) yogurt or kefir, ½ cup (125 mL) cottage or ricotta cheese, 1½ oz. (45 g) cheese.

Also:

2 to 3 tbsp. (30 to 45 mL) unsaturated vegetable oils or soft margarines that are low in saturated fats.

The Big Four: Vegetarian Nutrition in a Nutshell

OK, so you've decided to become a vegetarian. You have your reasons. Fine. No one (except possibly your Aunt Gertrude) will argue with you about such personal things as your moral convictions regarding the sanctity of life or your belief in the spiritual oneness of the universe. But when it comes to the nutritional aspects of your vegetarian diet, you'd darn well better know what you're doing. It isn't hard. It just takes a little planning.

A healthy lacto-ovo vegetarian diet is not only perfectly reasonable, it's also fairly easy to follow. Nutritionally speaking, the main issues are protein, iron, vitamin B12 and calcium. These are the Big Four. These are what Aunt Gertrude is concerned about. And, frankly, you should be too. Here's what you need to know in a nutshell (okay, a coconut shell).

1. Protein – essential for growth, tissue repair, and to help fight against infections.

This is the biggie, isn't it? How (on earth) will you (ever) get enough protein if you're not eating meat (for goodness sake, dear)? Well, it just so happens that meat isn't the only food that contains protein. A responsible (key word!) lacto-ovo vegetarian should have no problem obtaining adequate protein from a diet that includes a wide variety of foods: eggs, dairy products and legumes. If you are consuming enough calories to meet your energy needs, and assuming you do not depend solely on high-fat dairy products as your protein source, you can relax and eat your bean sprouts in peace. And don't obsess over combining all your nutrients at the same meal. Instead, look at your total diet over the course of the whole day. Some whole-grain toast at breakfast, a bean salad at lunch, a slice of cheese, a scrambled egg once in a while, a little tofu and you'll be doing just fine (so relax, Aunt Gertrude).

Protein Sources:
- Legumes (beans, peas and lentils)
- Soy foods (soybeans, tofu, tempeh, textured vegetable protein [TVP] and soy milk products)
- Peanut butter
- Seitan (wheat gluten)
- Nuts and seeds
- Grain products (wheat, rice, corn, barley, oats, millet, quinoa)
- Dairy products (milk, cheese, yogurt)
- Eggs

2. Iron - important for forming red blood cells.

The iron in plant foods and eggs is different from the type of iron found in red meat. It's there, it's just a bit harder to get at than the iron in red meats. In fact, vegetarian diets are often higher in total iron content than non-vegetarian diets, but the type of iron found in plant-based foods is poorly absorbed by the body. One thing that helps the body absorb this iron, however, is vitamin C. And that's the good news because a vegetarian diet tends to have plenty of vitamin C, which helps to unlock iron and make it available to the body. So what does this mean to you? It means that you should choose foods that are a good source of iron and make sure you're getting plenty of vitamin C as well. If all else fails, have a tall glass of orange juice with your oatmeal.

Iron Sources:
- Eggs
- Whole grains
- Dark green and leafy vegetables (broccoli, kale, peas, string beans, chard, spinach)
- Legumes (beans, lentils)
- Soy foods (soybeans, tofu, tempeh, TVP, soy milk products)
- Nuts and seeds (especially tahini [sesame paste] and almond butter)
- Dried fruits (raisins, apricots, figs)
- Blackstrap molasses

3. B12 — needed to form red blood cells and a healthy nervous system.

Other nutrients to think (but not obsess) about

Zinc, which can be found in chickpeas and lentils, as well as other legumes, sesame seeds, nuts, firm tofu, peanuts, wheat germ, milk products and eggs.

Vitamin D, which is available in fortified milk products, eggs and (yippee!) sunlight. So go outside once in a while.

Riboflavin, which is found in milk and eggs as well as soybeans, almonds, enriched cereals and nutritional yeast. It is also found, oddly, in mushrooms and sweet potatoes. Not to mention green leafy vegetables, dried fruits and whole-grain products.

A healthy lacto-ovo vegetarian diet, a diet that includes dairy products and eggs, will usually provide adequate amounts of vitamin B12. Since this nutrient is primarily found in animal products, only vegans need to make a special effort to obtain B12 from alternate sources, such as fortified soy products and beverages and certain breakfast cereals. You can also use Red Star nutritional yeast, which is a pleasantly cheesy-tasting powder that can be sprinkled on salads, cooked grains or even on popcorn. It is recommended that vegans have their blood levels of vitamin B12 checked annually by a physician to see if any additional supplements are necessary.

B12 sources:
- Dairy products (milk, cheese, yogurt)
- Fortified non-dairy beverages
- Fortified cereals
- Fortified meat alternatives like TVP and veggie burgers
- Nutritional yeast (Red Star brand in particular)

4. Calcium – essential for teeth, bones and healthy muscle function.

Calcium? No problem. If you're a lacto-ovo vegetarian and you include dairy products in your diet, you should be laughing, calciumwise. Milk, cheese and yogurt practically scream calcium. And if you also eat plenty of dark green vegetables (and why wouldn't you?), some tofu or fortified non-dairy milk and nibble the odd almond once in a while, you will be getting enough calcium.

Calcium sources:
- Dairy products (milk, cheese, yogurt)
- Fortified non-dairy beverages
- Fortified orange juice
- Dark green vegetables (broccoli, kale, bok choy)
- Dried figs
- Almonds
- Legumes (beans and lentils)
- Soy foods (especially tofu fortified with calcium)

How to Eat Out

You really hate to make a spectacle of yourself. But for a vegetarian, eating out at a restaurant presents a challenge. Fortunately, there are more vegetarian choices on restaurant menus now than ever before, so it may not be difficult to find something you can eat. Now take a deep breath and have a close look at the menu. How about:

- Pizza (easy one).

- Pasta with veggie or dairy-based sauce.

- Veggie burgers or falafel.

- A bagel with cream cheese and a salad or an egg salad plate.

- Bean burritos or tacos (ask if the refried beans are made with vegetable shortening).

- Veggie or cheese sandwich — anything from a grilled vegetable panini to a meatless sub sandwich from a fast-food place.

- Order a baked potato (or two) with vegetarian toppings.

- Have a huge salad, some good bread and dessert! If it's a Caesar salad, make sure you ask them to leave out the bacon bits and anchovies.

- Go Indian — always lots of vegetarian choices.

- Try Chinese or Thai, but ask if there's any meat or fish in the dishes you choose. Remember that many Asian dishes are made with oyster or fish sauce or a meat-based stock and that sometimes vegetables are "seasoned" with pork. Go for tofu or vegetarian vegetable dishes and plain steamed rice. Soups are often made with meat stock. Ask questions before ordering.

- Make dinner out of appetizers: bruschetta, rice-stuffed grape leaves, nachos with guacamole, fried zucchini sticks and dip, stuffed potato skins, antipasto without meat.

- Have an omelet or frittata, heavy on the vegetables.

- Check out a kosher dairy restaurant for cheese blintzes, potato latkes and veggie knishes.

Essential Supplies for the Vegetarian Kitchen

This is a wish list. You won't have all these things in your home all the time. Or even half the time. But let's say you did. Well, then you could make almost everything in this whole book at a moment's notice. Now wouldn't that be nice?

The Top 10

If you were planning to get stranded on a desert island with nothing but a swimsuit, a can opener and 10 food items, here's what you should pack. Oh, and by the way, don't forget your sunscreen.

- Rice
- Pasta
- Vegetable oil or olive oil
- Canned beans
- Tofu
- Peanut butter
- Canned tomatoes
- Onions
- Soy sauce
- Chocolate (hey, even a vegetarian cast-away needs a little treat once in a while)

Pantry Staples

Canned and dry beans (several kinds, such as red kidney beans, black beans, chickpeas, white kidney beans, pinto beans)
Canned tomatoes
Canned spaghetti sauce (the best you can afford)
Vegetable oil (canola, corn, soy, peanut or sunflower)
Olive oil (yes, yes, yes)
Vinegar (balsamic along with apple cider, wine or rice vinegar)
Soy sauce
Sesame oil
Peanut butter
Tahini
Vegetable stock (carton or can or bouillon cubes or powder)
Several kinds of pasta
Rice (white and brown)
Cornmeal
Couscous
Quinoa
Bulgur wheat
Rolled oats
TVP (textured vegetable protein)
Flour (white and whole wheat)
Cornstarch
Raisins or dried cranberries
Sun-dried tomatoes
Bread crumbs
Nuts (peanuts, almonds, walnuts, pine nuts)
Sesame seeds

Spices

Salt
Black pepper
Oregano
Basil
Cumin
Turmeric
Curry powder
Cayenne pepper
Crushed red pepper flakes
Cinnamon
Garam masala
Mexican chili powder

Fresh Stuff

Tofu (regular and/or extra firm)
Eggs
Milk
Yogurt
Onions
Garlic
Potatoes
Sweet potatoes
Fresh parsley
Cabbage
Carrots
Green and/or red sweet peppers
Mushrooms
Broccoli
Eggplant

Lettuce (romaine, iceberg, leaf,
    arugula or mixed baby greens)
Green beans
Winter squash (butternut,
    hubbard or acorn)
Zucchini
Breads (several kinds, such as
    sandwich bread, tortillas, pita
    and bagels)
Cheeses (Parmesan, cheddar,
    mozzarella, Monterey Jack,
    Swiss, feta, goat cheese)

And in the Freezer

Peas
Corn

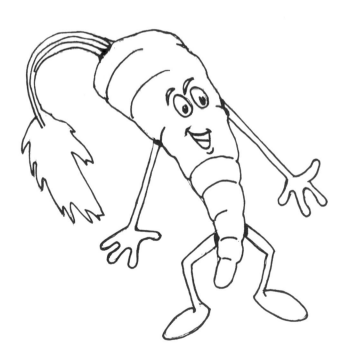

How to Vegetarianize a Recipe

No one would suggest that it is possible to create a vegetarian version of, say, roast beef (although, sadly, some have tried). But in many cases you can create wonderful vegetarian versions of meat-based favorites or adapt a new non-vegetarian recipe by eliminating the meat and making some clever substitions. Here are a few hints to get you started:

★ Identify the problematic components in the recipe. Is meat the lead player or does it just have a supporting role? Attempting to reproduce something like roast turkey, for instance, is a desperate and often disappointing endeavor. However, if the meat plays a secondary role to any vegetables or a sauce, you may be able to retain the integrity of the dish just by juggling or eliminating ingredients.

★ A flavorful vegetable stock can almost always be used in place of beef or chicken stock in a recipe. Buy prepared vegetable stock (carton, canned or bouillon cubes or powder) or make your own (see page 39).

★ Instead of ground beef, substitute a similar volume of rehydrated textured vegetable protein (TVP), crumbled frozen and defrosted tofu, mashed tempeh or commercial vegetarian "ground beef." Increase the other flavorings in the dish to compensate for the relative blandness of these meat stand-ins.

★ Experiment with the chunk form of TVP (which looks like dog kibble) in place of chunks of chicken or beef in stewy concoctions. Or use cubes of firm tofu or steamed tempeh.

★ Seitan (wheat gluten) can be used in place of sliced meat in a stir-fry or sauced dish. It has a very meat-like texture and blends unobtrusively into whatever else is going on.

★ It may be possible to eliminate the meat from a dish altogether without any adjustment whatsoever, or you can often just increase the amount of vegetables to make up for the missing meat.

★ Try eggplant or mushrooms instead of meat. Either one can provide a chewy, meaty texture that will more than compensate for whatever you took out.

★ Beans or lentils have a satisfyingly meaty quality that can add that certain something to a vegetarian dish. Bulgur wheat or cooked brown rice can also provide a nice, chewy texture.

★ Vegans can replace milk with plain soy, rice or almond non-dairy milk with practically no detectable difference in most recipes. Soy cheese can sometimes take the place of regular cheese as well (but success will vary with the type of product — experiment).

★ If all else fails, try imitation meat. These products, made to resemble ground beef, pepperoni, hot dogs or hamburgers, are widely available and can stand in for meat in most recipes and will do the job if you're really feeling deprived.

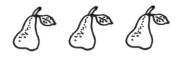

2. Appetizers, Snacks and Starters

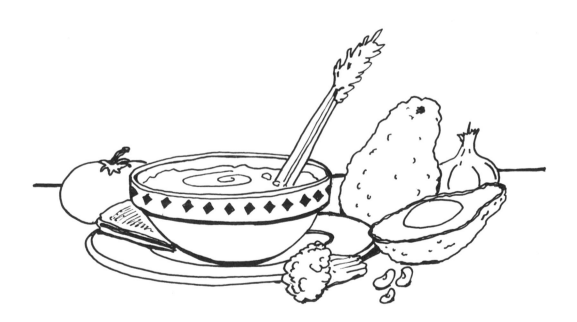

Hummus

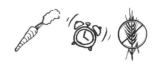

Ridiculously easy, absurdly cheap and absolutely delicious — this recipe makes a fresh, lemony hummus. Adjust the amounts of lemon and garlic to suit your taste.

1 (19 oz.)	1 (540 mL)	can chickpeas, drain and save the liquid (2 cups/500 mL cooked dried beans)
¼ cup	60 mL	tahini (see below or box) or, if unavailable, peanut butter
¼ cup	60 mL	lemon juice
2		cloves garlic, minced or pressed
½ tsp.	2 mL	ground cumin, if desired
½ tsp.	2 mL	salt
		parsley, chopped, for garnish
		olive oil, for garnish

Place the chickpeas, tahini, lemon juice, garlic, cumin and salt into the container of a blender or food processor and blend until the mixture is very smooth. Scrape down the sides several times adding as much liquid from the beans as is needed to make a smooth puree.

Taste and adjust the seasoning, if desired. Ideally, hummus should be a little thicker than sour cream. If it's too thick, add some additional liquid from the beans and blend again.

To serve, spread the hummus out in a shallow bowl, sprinkle with some chopped parsley and drizzle the top with a bit of olive oil. Serve with triangles of warmed pita bread for dipping.

Makes about 2 cups (500 mL).

Tahini

Tahini is a finely ground paste made from sesame seeds — sort of a Middle Eastern version of peanut butter. But instead of being used as a sandwich spread, tahini is a multipurpose ingredient that may be thinned and used as a sauce or added to a dish as a flavoring. In some recipes it may be possible to substitute peanut butter, but the flavor will be different. It is available in Middle Eastern grocery stores and most large supermarkets.

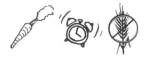

Chunky Guacamole

Chunks of avocado, tomato and onion allow the flavors of the ingredients in this popular dip to really stand out. Warning: no matter how much of this you make, you won't have enough.

2		medium size, ripe avocados
1		small red onion, finely chopped
2 tbsp.	30 mL	lime juice
1		medium tomato, seeded and finely chopped
1		fresh jalapeño pepper, seeded and finely chopped
¼ cup	60 mL	cilantro, chopped
½ tsp.	2 mL	salt

Cut the avocados in half, remove and discard the seeds and peel them. If they are ripe, the skin should come off easily. Dice the avocado flesh and dump it into a bowl.

Add the onion, tomato, jalapeño, cilantro, lime juice and salt, and toss, without mashing, to combine. The ingredients should remain separate and the mixture chunky.

Serve with tortilla chips for dipping or as an accompaniment to tacos, burritos or quesadillas.

Makes about 2 cups (500 mL).

Avocados

Most avocados are picked while they're still unripe and only begin to soften once they're off the tree. Like in your kitchen, for instance. Just leave a hard avocado at room temperature until it yields to pressure when you (very, very gently) squeeze it in your hand. You can try to hurry this process by placing it in a paper bag with an apple. Apples emit a gas (really!) that helps other fruit to ripen. But whatever you do, don't refrigerate an avocado before it's soft or it will never ripen properly.

Special Bonus Project!

A Beautiful Avocado Plant for (Almost) Free

No! Stop! Don't throw out that avocado seed! It would be like, well, murder. Let it grow into a plant instead. Here's how you do it.

First, peel off as much of the brown outer skin as you can easily remove from the seed. Now determine which end is up. (The bottom of the seed will be more flattened; the top will be more pointy.) Next, poke three toothpicks around the "equator" of the seed, roughly equidistant from each other. Use these toothpicks to support the seed (bottom-side-down) over the opening of a wide-mouthed jar (like an old mayonnaise or jam jar). Fill the jar with enough water to come about halfway up the sides of the avocado seed, at least to the level of the toothpicks, and place the jar in a sunny spot. Now wait. For how long? Who knows. Probably weeks. Replace the water as it evaporates and be very patient.

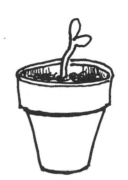

The first thing you will see is a root sprouting out from the bottom of the seed. This root will reach down into the water. Then, eventually, a shoot will appear at the top of the seed, then some leaves. At this point, you can plant the seed in a flowerpot filled with potting soil. Keep it on a sunny windowsill, water it regularly and you now have a lovely plant.

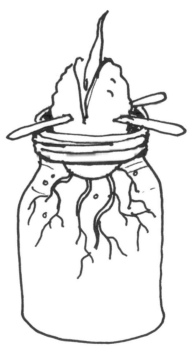

In 20 years, it may even produce an avocado.

Fresh Tomato Salsa

Sure, you can buy salsa by the vat in any supermarket, but it won't taste like this. Fresh salsa, especially when tomatoes are in season, is something else altogether. Try it.

1 lb.	500 g	perfectly ripe plum tomatoes (about 4 medium)
½		medium red onion, finely chopped
2		cloves garlic, minced or pressed
1 or 2		fresh jalapeño peppers, seeded and minced, or more (go ahead, be wild and crazy)
¼ cup	60 mL	cilantro, chopped
2 tbsp.	30 mL	lime juice
1 tsp.	5 mL	salt

Cut the tomatoes in half crosswise and gently squeeze out as much of the juicy, seedy pulp as you can and discard it. Chop the tomatoes finely (but don't pulverize them) and place in a bowl.

Add the onion, garlic, jalapeños, cilantro, lime juice and salt. Taste and adjust the seasoning, if desired. This is not a scientific formula. You can add and subtract to your heart's content.

Let salsa sit, at room temperature, for about 30 minutes to allow the flavors to blend before serving.

Is that great, or what?

Makes about 3 cups (750 mL).

How to Chop an Onion Without Really Crying

Method #1:
Place the onion on a cutting board. Set the cutting board on the front burner of your stove. *Do not turn on the burner!* Now turn the back burner on to medium heat and chop to your heart's content. The heat somehow magically draws the onion fumes away from you, leaving you free to chop tearlessly. Really. (Remember to turn off the back burner when you're done.)

Method #2:
Wear contact lenses.

Method #3:
Wear a diving mask.

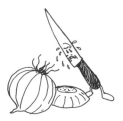

Speedy Breakfast Burrito

Yikes! You're late! But you're hungry. Quick! Make this and run.

Scramble an egg or two or make some scrambled tofu (see page 88) and scoop it onto a fresh tortilla. (If you have an extra 20 seconds, zap the tortilla in the microwave to warm it first.) Slop on a couple of spoonfuls of fresh tomato salsa, sprinkle some shredded cheese on top, fold up the bottom, roll in the sides and eat.

Now get out of here!

Spicy Black Bean Dip

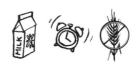

This is one of the fastest dips around, both coming and going.
It takes about three minutes to make and only a little longer to
disappear.

1 (19 oz.)	1 (540 mL)	can black beans, drained (or 2 cups/500 mL cooked dried beans)
½ cup	125 mL	tomato salsa, homemade or store-bought (mild, medium or whatever)
1		clove garlic, minced or pressed
2 tbsp.	30 mL	cilantro, chopped, if desired (for cilantro-lovers)
		sour cream, for garnish
		shredded cheese, for garnish

Dump the beans, salsa, garlic and cilantro into the container of a blender
or food processor and blend until combined but not totally smooth.
For more texture (and less stuff to clean up), mash the beans in a bowl
with a potato masher or a fork, then stir in the salsa, garlic and chopped
cilantro. Your choice.

Scoop the bean mixture into a bowl, top with a dollop of sour cream
and sprinkle with some shredded cheese (and more cilantro, if you have it).

Serve with tortilla chips or vegetable dippers.

Makes about 2½ cups (625 mL).

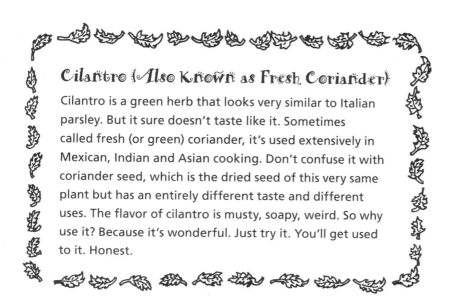

Cilantro (Also Known as Fresh Coriander)

Cilantro is a green herb that looks very similar to Italian
parsley. But it sure doesn't taste like it. Sometimes
called fresh (or green) coriander, it's used extensively in
Mexican, Indian and Asian cooking. Don't confuse it with
coriander seed, which is the dried seed of this very same
plant but has an entirely different taste and different
uses. The flavor of cilantro is musty, soapy, weird. So why
use it? Because it's wonderful. Just try it. You'll get used
to it. Honest.

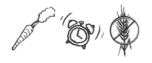

Tomato Bruschetta Topping

Best made with flavorful, in-season tomatoes and fresh basil, you'll think of a dozen different ways to use it. Perfect, of course, as an appetizer on toasted Italian bread, but also delicious spooned into an omelet or tossed with pasta.

3		perfectly ripe medium-sized tomatoes, finely chopped
2		cloves garlic, minced or pressed
2 tbsp.	30 mL	fresh basil, chopped
1 tsp.	5 mL	salt
¼ tsp.	1 mL	black pepper

In a bowl, mix together the tomatoes, garlic, basil, salt and pepper. Let the mixture sit for at least 10 minutes at room temperature before serving.

Makes about 1½ cups (375 mL).

Tzatziki

The secret to making a great, creamy tzatziki is to drain the excess liquid out of both the yogurt and the cucumber. This will give you a thick, delicious dip that is fresher tasting than anything you can buy ready-made.

3 cups	750 mL	plain, natural yogurt, without additives or thickeners (or see Greek Yogurt, left)
1		seedless English cucumber
1 tsp.	5 mL	salt
1		clove garlic, minced or pressed
1 tbsp.	15 mL	fresh mint, dill or chives (or a mixture), chopped
¼ tsp.	1 mL	black pepper

First, drain the excess liquid from the yogurt, unless you're using Greek-style yogurt (see note below). The easiest way to do this is to take a paper coffee filter, place it into a filter holder or strainer over a bowl or measuring cup and dump the yogurt into the filter to drain. If you don't have such equipment, simply spoon the yogurt into a strainer lined with

Greek Yogurt

Greek-style yogurt is yogurt that has already been drained to thicken it. So if you're able to get it, you can skip the draining step in this recipe. Reduce the amount of yogurt to 1½ cups (375 mL) and and mix it with the drained cucumber and other ingredients without further messing around.

a clean paper towel and place it over a bowl to catch the liquid. Either way, let the yogurt drain, refrigerated, for at least 2 hours or as long as overnight. The longer you drain the yogurt, the thicker it will become.

When the yogurt is drained and ready to use, scrub the cucumber and grate it on the coarse holes of a grater or with the shredding blade of a food processor.

Place the shredded cucumber into a bowl, sprinkle with the salt and let sit for about 1 hour to allow the salt to draw out the excess liquid.

After the hour, drain the shredded cucumber thoroughly and, if you want to be really fanatical about this, squeeze the remaining water out by hand.

Place the drained cucumber in a bowl. Stir in the drained yogurt, garlic and chopped mint or other herbs. Taste and adjust the seasoning with black pepper and additional salt, if desired.

Ta da! Your very own delicious homemade tzatziki is ready to serve as a dip with pita bread or fresh vegetables or as an accompaniment to grilled vegetables.

Makes about 2½ cups (625 mL).

Baba Ghanoush

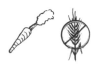

Adjust the amount of garlic to suit your taste; this recipe makes a medium-garlicky dip. You can even use roasted garlic (see page 27) instead of raw garlic for a mellower flavor.

1		medium eggplant
¼ cup	60 mL	tahini
¼ cup	60 mL	lemon juice
2		cloves garlic, minced or pressed
1 tbsp.	15 mL	olive oil
1 tsp.	5 mL	salt

Preheat the oven to 450°F (230°C) or preheat the barbecue grill on high.

Prick the eggplant all over with a fork (this is necessary to avoid explosion), place on a baking pan in the preheated oven and bake for about 1 hour, turning over after 30 minutes, until the skin is blackened and the insides are soft. If you're using a barbecue, place the eggplant on a foil pan on the grill, cover and cook, turning once or twice, until it is charred and soft, about 30 to 40 minutes. The barbecue method will produce a smokier taste that, in this case, is an excellent thing, but either way is fine.

Let the blackened eggplant cool just until you can handle it, then cut in half and scoop the pulp out into a bowl. Mash it roughly with a fork.

Add the tahini, lemon juice, garlic, olive oil and salt to the eggplant and mix well with the fork. This can be done in a food processor, if you prefer a smoother dip, but be careful not to overprocess the mixture — it should retain a little texture.

Spoon the baba ghanoush into a bowl and serve with pita bread or vegetable dippers.

Makes about 2 cups (500 mL).

Eggplant Caviar

Serve a scoop of this on a bed of lettuce as a first course or spoon it into a bowl and serve it as a dip with pita chips or hearty rye bread. Delicious, dark and handsome.

1		medium eggplant
2 tbsp.	30 mL	olive oil or vegetable oil
1		medium onion, chopped
2		cloves garlic, minced or pressed
1		medium green or red sweet pepper, chopped
2 tbsp.	30 mL	tomato paste
1 tbsp.	15 mL	honey or brown sugar
1 tsp.	5 mL	salt
½ tsp.	2 mL	black pepper
2 tbsp.	30 mL	lemon juice

Preheat the oven to 450°F (230°C) or preheat the barbecue grill on high.

Prick the eggplant all over with a fork (this is necessary to avoid explosion), place on a baking pan in the preheated oven and bake for about 1 hour, turning over after 30 minutes, until the skin is blackened and the insides are soft. If you're using a barbecue, place the eggplant on a foil pan on the grill, cover and cook, turning once or twice, until charred and soft, about 30 to 40 minutes. The barbecue method will produce a smokier taste — excellent — but either method is fine.

Let the blackened eggplant cool just until you can handle it, then cut in half and scoop the pulp out into a bowl. Mash it roughly with a fork.

While the eggplant is cooking, heat the oil in a medium skillet over medium heat. Add the onion and cook, stirring, for 8 to 10 minutes, until soft.

Eggplant

Resist, if you possibly can, buying the hugest eggplant monstrosity at the market. Giant eggplants can be bitter and seedy; small to medium ones will have better flavor and texture.

Look for a firm eggplant with shiny skin and with no bruises or brown spots. The most familiar type is the bulbous purple-black type of eggplant. These are useful when you want meaty slices or chunks or to roast whole for a dip. Long, thin Asian eggplants are best to use in a stir-fry or vegetable stew or to slice in half lengthwise for the grill.

Add the garlic and sweet pepper, lower the heat to medium-low and continue to cook for another 8 to 10 minutes, stirring occasionally.

Stir in the tomato paste, honey or brown sugar, salt and pepper and cook for just a minute or two to combine the flavors.

Add the mashed eggplant pulp to the mixture in the pan and cook the mixture for about 5 minutes, stirring often.

Remove from the heat, stir in the lemon juice and place in the refrigerator to chill before serving.

Taste and adjust seasoning, if necessary, when cool.

Serve the eggplant caviar with crackers, bread or pita triangles.

Makes about 2 cups (500 mL).

Roasted Garlic

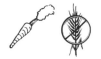

Of course, you can roast just a single head of garlic, but while you're at it, why not do a whole bunch? Once you've tasted what roasting can do for raw garlic, you'll find a zillion ways to use it. You can serve a whole head as an appetizer (see sidebar) or squish out the pulp and use it to season salad dressings, dips or mashed potatoes. Roasting transforms raw garlic from a wild and uncivilized maniac into an affable, mellow eccentric. Sort of like when your Uncle Chuckie got married.

4		whole heads of garlic
1 tbsp.	15 mL	olive oil or vegetable oil
¼ cup	60 mL	vegetable stock or water
¼ tsp.	1 mL	salt

Preheat the oven to 375°F (190°C).

Gently remove any excess papery skin from the garlic, without breaking up the heads or peeling them completely.

With a sharp knife, cut a thin slice from the top (the pointy end) of each head, just to slightly expose the innards of the cloves. Arrange the garlic heads cut side up in a small baking dish and drizzle with the oil. Pour the vegetable stock or water into the bottom of the dish, sprinkle the garlic heads with the salt and cover.

Place in the preheated oven and bake for 45 minutes to 1 hour, uncovering the dish for the last 10 minutes of baking time to allow the garlic to brown.

That's all. Now, go and have your way with it.

Roasted Garlic With Goat Cheese The Best Appetizer Ever

Roast one head of garlic for each person you're serving. Place a head of roasted garlic on a plate, along with a scoop of goat cheese and some crusty French bread.

Smear goat cheese on the bread, squish out a clove of garlic on top and eat.

Am I right?

Mexican Meltdown

This wonderfully gloppy, cheesy goop will make you instantly famous. Be prepared to make it for every party.

2 tbsp.	30 mL	olive oil
4		green onions, chopped
2 to 3		jalapeño peppers, chopped
1		medium onion, chopped
½		medium red sweet pepper, chopped
1 cup	250 mL	diced tomato, canned or fresh (about 2 medium)
2		cloves garlic, minced or pressed
½ tsp.	2 mL	salt
¼ tsp.	1 mL	black pepper
¼ cup	60 mL	heavy or whipping cream (30 to 40%)
4 cups	1 L	shredded cheddar or Monterey Jack cheese
2 tbsp.	30 mL	all-purpose flour
1 tsp.	5 mL	ground cumin

Heat the olive oil in a large skillet over medium heat. Add the green onions, jalapeños, onion and red pepper and cook, stirring, until vegetables are soft, about 6 to 8 minutes.

Stir in the tomatoes, garlic, salt and pepper and let simmer for 5 minutes, until the tomatoes are softened.

Stir in the cream.

In a bowl, toss the cheese with the flour and cumin. Add to the tomato mixture in the skillet and cook just long enough to melt the cheese.

Transfer to a bowl or serve directly from the skillet with tortilla chips for dipping.

Gooey deliciousness.

Serves 6 to 8 as an appetizer.

Cheese

Use whatever cheese you happen to have. The recipe calls for cheddar and all you have is Swiss? Use it. The taste will be different but, who knows, you may even like it better. Rule of thumb: when substituting a cheese, try to substitute with a cheese of the same consistency (soft, medium or hard).

Veggie Pâté

This spread looks (and even tastes) so much like liver pâté that it almost feels like cheating. Serve it with crackers or thinly sliced French bread and let everyone wonder if you've started eating meat again.

3 tbsp.	45 mL	olive oil or vegetable oil
2		medium onions, chopped
1 (19 oz)	1 (540 mL)	can lentils, drained (or 2 cups/500 mL cooked dried lentils)
4		hard-boiled eggs, peeled (see page 83)
1 tbsp.	15 mL	peanut butter
½ tsp.	2 mL	salt
¼ tsp.	1 mL	black pepper

Heat the oil in a small skillet over medium heat. Add the chopped onions and cook, stirring often, for 10 to 12 minutes, until the onions are golden brown. Remove from heat and set aside.

If you have a food processor, dump the sautéed onions, lentils and the hard-boiled eggs into the container and process until the mixture is finely chopped but not totally smooth. Add the peanut butter, salt and pepper. Process until blended and creamy. If you don't have a food processor, chop the ingredients as finely as possible then, using a fork or potato masher, mash everything together in a bowl until the paté is as smooth as you can get it. The fork method will leave the mixture rougher in texture but still delicious.

Pack the paté into a bowl or small soufflé dish, cover and chill. Serve with bread or crackers.

Makes about 3 cups (750 mL).

Pseudo-Hollandaise Sauce

Use this as a dipping sauce for cooked artichokes (see below) or spoon it over freshly steamed broccoli or asparagus. Terribly elegant, very delicious, ridiculously easy.

2		eggs
2 tbsp.	30 mL	lemon juice
¼ tsp.	1 mL	salt
1 cup	250 mL	butter

Place the eggs, lemon juice and salt in the container of a blender.

In a small saucepan, bring the butter to a boil over medium heat. Remove from the heat and, with the blender running, pour the hot butter in a stream through the small opening in the blender's lid. Blend until the sauce is thickened and smooth. Serve immediately.

Makes about 2 cups (500 mL).

Artichokes: The Porcupines of the Vegetable World

For a fun appetizer, buy one large fresh artichoke per person. With scissors, snip off the prickly tip of each leaf and remove any discolored leaves. Trim the stem so the artichoke has a flat bottom. Arrange the artichokes in a steamer basket over boiling water and steam for 30 to 45 minutes, until you can easily pull out a leaf. Place the artichokes on serving plates and serve warm with Pseudo-Hollandaise Sauce (above), or chill and serve cold with Basic Vinaigrette Dressing (page 76).

To eat, remove the leaves one at a time. Dip the base of each leaf into the dipping sauce and scrape it between your teeth to remove the soft fleshy part of the leaf along with the sauce. Discard the fibrous bit that's left over. Continue removing leaves until you get to the fuzzy middle, or "choke," — this is the heart of the artichoke. Scrape the furry bit off and eat the delicious bottom.

There. Don't you feel sophisticated?

Do-It-Yourself Vegetarian Sushi Rolls

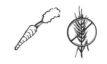

No really, you can do this. They're easy and fun to make and, seriously, the best party food ever. You can find everything you need at Asian grocery stores and in many large supermarkets.

First make the sushi rice:

2 cups	500 mL	uncooked Japanese sushi rice
2½ cups	625 mL	water
¼ cup	60 mL	Japanese rice vinegar
2 tbsp.	30 mL	sugar
½ tsp.	2 mL	salt

Place the rice in a bowl and rinse well in several changes of water until the water is no longer cloudy. Drain thoroughly in a strainer.

In a medium saucepan, combine the rice and water and bring to a boil over high heat.

Stir once, reduce the heat to low, then cover the pan and let cook for about 15 minutes or until all the water is absorbed and the rice is tender but not mushy. Dump the rice into a large bowl.

In a small bowl, stir together the rice vinegar, sugar and salt until the sugar is dissolved. Pour over the cooked rice and mix together gently. Don't scramble the rice; just combine so the rice is evenly coated with the vinegar mixture.

Let cool to room temperature while you prepare the rest of the ingredients for your sushi rolls.

To assemble:

1	medium carrot, peeled and cut into very thin lengthwise matchsticks
1	ripe avocado, peeled, pitted and cut into thin slivers
4	green onions, trimmed and cut into lengthwise slivers
½	seedless English cucumber, cut into very thin lengthwise matchsticks
½	small red or yellow sweet pepper, cut into lengthwise slivers
6	sheets Japanese nori seaweed
	bamboo mat for rolling the sushi
	prepared Japanese wasabi horseradish (sold in tubes)
	soy sauce for dipping (a gluten-free brand, if desired)

Arrange all the filling ingredients on a plate on your work surface.

Place the sushi mat (with the slats running crosswise) in front of you on your work surface and lay a sheet of nori seaweed, shiny-side down, on the mat.

With moistened fingers, press about one-sixth of the rice onto the sheet of nori, leaving about 1 inch (2 cm) uncovered at the end farthest away from you. Pat it down evenly.

Now the fillings. Choose three or four filling ingredients to start and arrange them sparingly and crosswise over the rice, starting about 1 inch (2 cm) from the edge nearest to you and leaving about 1 inch (2 cm) of rice uncovered at the far end. (Arranging the fillings this way will give you a sort of spiral effect. If you want all the fillings in the *middle* of the roll, make a row of filling ingredients crosswise about ½ inch (2 cm) from the edge closest to you, rather than spreading them out over the entire surface of the rice.)

Pat the fillings down gently.

With a finger, moisten the uncovered nori (at the far end) with a bit of water.

Now to roll the thing up. Starting at the edge closest to you, tightly roll up the nori, rice and fillings, using the mat to help tighten the roll as you go along. When you get to the end, stick the roll shut with the moistened end of the nori and roll the mat firmly to seal.

Transfer the roll to a plate or tray and cover with plastic wrap.

Repeat with the remaining rice, nori and filling ingredients. Choose different combinations of vegetables to vary the rolls.

After everything is rolled up, cut each roll crosswise into eight pieces with a sharp knife.

Arrange on a platter and serve with wasabi and soy sauce for dipping. Take a bow.

Makes 48 pieces.

Salsa Cheese Squares

This great munchie can be thrown together in minutes with stuff you probably already have in your fridge and pantry. For a spicier version of this recipe, substitute chopped fresh jalapeño peppers for all or part of the canned green chiles.

2 cups	500 mL	shredded cheddar cheese
2 cups	500 mL	shredded Monterey Jack cheese
2 (4.5 oz)	2 (127 mL)	cans chopped green chiles
1 cup	250 mL	biscuit mix, homemade (see page 194) or store-bought
4		eggs, beaten
½ cup	125 mL	milk
½ cup	125 mL	prepared tomato salsa, any kind

Preheat the oven to 425°F (220°C). Grease a 9 × 13–inch (23 × 33 cm) rectangular baking dish.

Sprinkle the cheeses evenly over the bottom of the prepared baking dish. Spread the chiles evenly over the cheeses.

In a mixing bowl, beat together the biscuit mix, eggs and milk. Pour this mixture over the cheese and chiles, spreading it out to cover as much of the dish as possible.

Dollop the salsa on top of everything.

Place in the oven and bake for 25 to 30 minutes, until set. The mixture will be puffed and lightly browned in spots. Let cool for about 10 minutes before cutting into squares. Serve warm.

Makes about 25 squares.

Zucchini Bites

Too often the object of culinary derision, the poor, gentle zucchini doesn't deserve the scorn heaped upon it. This delicious and easy appetizer is guaranteed to convert even a hard-core zuke hater. No, really.

3 cups	750 mL	shredded zucchini (2 to 3 medium zukes)
4		eggs, beaten
1 cup	250 mL	biscuit mix, homemade (see page 194) or store-bought
½ cup	125 mL	grated Parmesan cheese
⅓ cup	75 mL	olive oil or vegetable oil
1		small onion, finely chopped
2 tbsp.	30 mL	fresh parsley, chopped
2 tbsp.	30 mL	fresh basil, chopped (or 2 tsp./10 mL dried)
½ tsp.	2 mL	hot pepper sauce, if you like that sort of thing
1 tsp.	5 mL	salt
¼ tsp.	1 mL	black pepper

Preheat the oven to 350°F (180°C). Grease a 9 × 13–inch (23 × 33 cm) rectangular baking dish.

In a large bowl, combine the zucchini, eggs, biscuit mix, Parmesan cheese, oil, onion, parsley, basil, hot pepper sauce, salt and pepper. Spread the mixture into the prepared baking dish.

Place in the preheated oven and bake for 25 to 30 minutes, until it's just beginning to brown lightly on top.

Let cool slightly, and then cut into squares (or diamonds or triangles or trapezoids) and serve hot or at room temperature. Let them just try and guess what's in it.

Makes at least 24 squares.

Quesadillas

Is it an appetizer? Is it a main dish? Who cares? It's fast, it's good, it's fun.

You'll definitely need:
Flour tortillas, large or small
Tomato salsa (store-bought or homemade (see page 22), any kind you like)
Shredded Monterey Jack or cheddar cheese

You may also want to add:

Refried beans, canned or homemade (see below)

Chopped jalapeño peppers, onions, sweet peppers, olives, mushrooms, tomatoes — whatever

Start with one flour tortilla.

If you're using refried beans, spread a layer of beans to within ½ inch (1 cm) of the edge of the tortilla.

Spoon the salsa over the beans, or just start with the salsa, then sprinkle with shredded cheese and any other ingredients you're using.

Slap a second tortilla on top, pressing down to squash the two sides together, like a sandwich.

Now heat a large frying pan or griddle over medium heat for a minute or two, until hot, without using any oil or other fat to grease the pan.

Place the tortilla sandwich in the pan and cook, squishing down lightly with a spatula, until the bottom begins to brown slightly. Flip the quesadilla over to allow the other side to brown slightly and the cheese inside to melt.

Remove to a cutting board and cut into wedges with a pizza cutter or sharp knife.

Repeat until you are full.

Do-It-Yourself Refried Beans

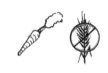

Make a double batch of these refried beans and keep them in the freezer to use in quesadillas or wherever you want to put them. If you want to go all the way and start with dry beans, see page 51.

1 tbsp.	15 mL	olive oil or vegetable oil
1		onion, chopped
1		clove garlic, minced or pressed
2 (19 oz)	2 (540 mL)	cans pinto or black beans (or 4 cups/1 L cooked dried beans)
½ tsp.	2 mL	salt, or to taste

In a large, heavy skillet, heat the oil over medium heat. Add the onion and garlic and cook, stirring, until the onion is quite soft, about 10 minutes.

Drain the canned beans (if you're using canned), but reserve the liquid. (If you're cooking dried beans, drain them before adding them to the skillet, but save some of the liquid.)

Add the beans to the pan and cook, stirring almost constantly and mashing them with a potato masher or a wooden spoon.

Add some of the liquid from the cans or bean-cooking water to the beans and continue to cook, stirring and mashing, until the mixture is thick and the beans are about half mashed. You can add more liquid (or water) to make the refried beans as runny or as thick as you like.

Serve sprinkled with cheese as a side dish with rice or tortillas, as a filling for burritos or as an ingredient in quesadillas or nachos.

Makes about 3 cups (750 mL).

Nacho-Stuffed Potato Shells

The perfect TV snack. Add a salad and it's dinner if you eat both halves.

4		large potatoes, scrubbed
1 cup	250 mL	store-bought tomato salsa, any kind
1 cup	250 mL	shredded Monterey Jack or Cheddar cheese

Bake the potatoes in the oven or microwave until completely soft inside (see page 175 for detailed instructions).

Let the potatoes cool slightly, then cut each in half lengthwise and carefully scoop most of the flesh out into a bowl, leaving about an ⅛-inch (0.25 cm) thick shell. (Save the flesh for another use, like mashed potatoes or to top a shepherd's pie).

Cut each potato shell in half lengthwise, making little canoe-shaped skins. Arrange flesh side up on a baking sheet.

Spoon a little salsa into each skin, and top with a mound of shredded cheese.

Bake for 10 minutes at 400°F (200°C), until the cheese is melted and bubbly. Yum.

Makes 16 stuffed potato wedges.

Muncho Grande Platter

Resistance is futile.

1 (19 oz.)	1 (540 mL)	can black or pinto beans (2 cups/500 mL cooked dried beans)
½ cup	125 mL	corn kernels, frozen or cut from a cooked cob
¼ cup	60 mL	red or yellow onion, chopped
1 or 2		jalapeño peppers, seeded and chopped
1		clove garlic, minced or pressed
2 tbsp.	30 mL	lime juice
1 tbsp.	15 mL	olive oil or vegetable oil
½ tsp.	2 mL	ground cumin
1 cup	250 mL	spreadable cream cheese (or 1 [8 oz/250 mL] package)
2		green onions, chopped
1		medium tomato, chopped
1		avocado, diced
½ cup	125 mL	shredded Monterey Jack or cheddar cheese

In a bowl, stir together the beans, corn, onion, jalapeños and garlic.

Add the lime juice, oil and cumin and stir to mix.

Cover and refrigerate for 1 to 2 hours, to allow the flavors to blend.

Just before serving, spread the cream cheese out onto a serving plate. Spoon the bean mixture over the top, and then sprinkle with the green onions, tomato, avocado and shredded cheese.

Serve with tortilla chips for dipping.

Serves 6 to 8 as an appetizer.

3. Soups from Scratch

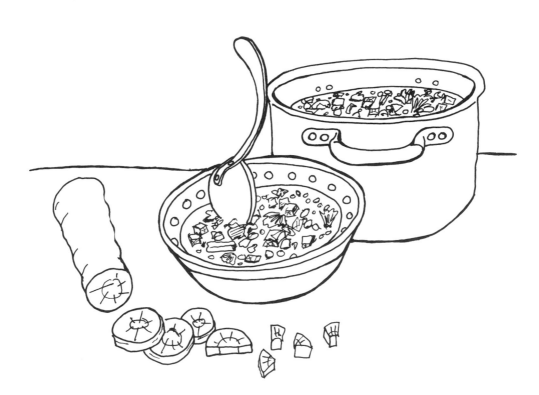

Golden Vegetable Stock

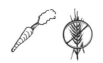

This cheerful golden stock can be used anytime you need a good, basic vegetable broth or stock or as a substitute for chicken stock in a recipe. Cook up a big batch and freeze it in small (2 cup/500 mL) containers so you'll always have some homemade stock ready to use when you need it.

4		medium carrots, cut into chunks
2		medium onions, cut into chunks
2		parsnips, cut into chunks
1		leek, carefully washed and sliced
1		head garlic, separated into cloves but not peeled
1 cup	250 mL	fresh parsley, roughly chopped
12 cups	3 L	water
1 tbsp.	15 mL	salt
1 tsp.	5 mL	turmeric (the secret ingredient!)
¼ tsp.	1 mL	or more, to taste, black pepper

Combine all the ingredients in a large pot or Dutch oven and bring to a boil over high heat.

Cover the pot, reduce the heat to low and let simmer for 1½ to 2 hours.

Taste and adjust seasoning, if necessary.

Let cool to room temperature before straining to remove the soggy vegetables.

Use the stock immediately or refrigerate or freeze for later use. Discard the sad vegetables or, better yet, add them to your compost bucket.

Makes about 10 cups (2.5 L).

Roasted Veggie Variation:

For a darker stock with a more robust flavor try this:

Toss the carrots, onions, parsnips, leek, and garlic with 1 tbsp. (15 mL) of olive oil in a large roasting pan. Place in the oven and bake at 400°F (200°C) for about 45 minutes, until the vegetables are beginning to brown and caramelize, stirring occasionally. Transfer the roasted vegetables to a stock pot. Pour 2 cups (500 mL) of the total amount of water in the recipe (above) into the roasting pan and stir to dissolve the brown bits that remain on the bottom of the pan. Add this to the stock pot along with all the other ingredients and continue the recipe as above.

The Stock Bag

Instead of throwing out all those vegetable trimmings (peels, tips, leaves, seedy innards) dump them into a bag and toss it into the freezer. You can continue to add to the bag whenever you have something to throw in and use it when you're ready to make a pot of stock. Brilliant.

Try:
- Scrubbed potato peels (but not the eyes or any green parts)
- Pea pods
- Onion ends (green parts too)
- Green or red pepper insides
- Celery leaves and bottoms
- Carrot peels
- Mushroom stems
- Wilted beans (or anything else that's wilted but not rotten)
- Mushy tomatoes

Split Pea Soup

You'd think that something like split pea soup would take hours to make, wouldn't you? It doesn't.

2 cups	500 mL	split peas (green or yellow, it doesn't matter)
8 cups	2 L	cold water
2		stalks celery, chopped
2		medium carrots, chopped
2		medium onions, chopped
1 tsp.	5 mL	salt
½ tsp.	2 mL	black pepper
2 tbsp.	30 mL	fresh parsley, chopped

Rinse the split peas in several changes of cold water, and then place them in a large saucepan or Dutch oven. Add the cold water and bring to a boil over medium-high heat.

Reduce the heat to low, cover the pot and simmer for about 20 minutes, stirring occasionally, until the peas are soft.

Add the celery, carrots, onions, salt, pepper and parsley. Bring the soup to a boil over medium-high heat, and then reduce the heat to low and simmer, covered, for another 30 minutes, until the vegetables are tender and the split peas have almost completely disintegrated.

Taste and adjust seasoning, if necessary.

Makes 6 to 8 servings.

Tomato and Chickpea Soup

A big bowl (or two) of this soup, a loaf of good bread and it's dinner. Well, okay, maybe just a sliver of apple pie and a small scoop of ice cream too...

2 tbsp.	30 mL	olive oil or vegetable oil
2		medium zucchinis, cut into ¼ inch (.5 cm) cubes
2		cloves garlic, minced or pressed
1		medium onion, chopped
1 (28 oz.)	1 (796 mL)	can diced tomatoes (or 3 cups/750 mL chopped fresh tomatoes)
1 tbsp.	15 mL	tomato paste
4 cups	1 L	vegetable stock, homemade or store-bought canned or from bouillon cubes or powder)
1 (19 oz.)	1 (540 mL)	can chickpeas, drained (or 2 cups/500 mL cooked dried beans)
1 (10 oz.)	1 (284 g)	package fresh spinach, washed and coarsely chopped (about 6 cups/1.5 L loose leaves)
1 tsp.	5 mL	salt
¼ tsp.	1 mL	black pepper
		grated Parmesan cheese, for sprinkling

Vegetable Stock

In any recipe that calls for vegetable stock, you may use your own homemade, prepared stock that comes in a can or carton or even good-quality bouillon cubes or powder. Keep in mind, however, that store-bought stocks tend to be saltier than homemade, so taste before adding additional salt to the recipe.

Heat the oil in a large pot or Dutch oven over medium heat. Add the zucchini, garlic and onion and cook, stirring, for 6 to 8 minutes, until the vegetables are just softened.

Add the tomatoes, tomato paste, vegetable stock and chickpeas. Bring to a boil, then reduce the heat to medium-low and simmer for 10 minutes.

Add the chopped spinach and let cook for a minute or two, until wilted.

Stir in the salt and pepper and serve with Parmesan cheese to sprinkle at the table.

Makes about 6 to 8 servings.

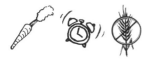

Quick Lentil Soup

A substantial soup in less than half an hour. You need this recipe.

1 tbsp.	15 mL	olive oil or vegetable oil
1		medium onion, chopped
2		cloves garlic, minced or pressed
1		medium carrot, chopped
1		stalk celery, chopped
1 tsp.	5 mL	ground cumin
1 (28 oz.)	1 (796 mL)	can diced tomatoes (or 3 cups/750 mL chopped fresh tomatoes)
1 (19 oz.)	1 (540 mL)	can lentils, drained (or 2 cups/500 mL cooked dried lentils)
1½ cups	375 mL	vegetable stock, homemade or store-bought (canned or from bouillon cubes or powder)
1 tsp.	5 mL	salt

Heat the oil in a large pot or Dutch oven over medium heat. Add the onion, garlic, carrot, celery and cumin and cook, stirring once in a while, for about 10 minutes, until the vegetables are softened.

Add the diced tomatoes, lentils, vegetable stock and salt and bring to a boil over medium-high heat.

Reduce the heat to low, cover the pot and let the soup simmer for about 15 minutes, until the vegetables are tender.

Adjust seasoning, if necessary, and serve. Done.

Makes 4 servings.

Tomatoes: A Slightly Complicated Business

A tomato is a tomato is a tomato, right? Well, not exactly. Sometimes it's best to buy fresh tomatoes for cooking; other times canned tomatoes are a better choice. It depends on the season and the recipe.

In summer, when tomatoes are in season, look for tomatoes that are firm but not as hard as a rock. They should have tight, shiny skin that is at least half red. Smell one. It should have a tomato aroma. Avoid squishy, overripe tomatoes unless they're super-cheap and you plan to use them immediately.

In winter you're usually better off using canned tomatoes for cooking purposes. They're available whole, diced or crushed and will have better flavor than those out-of-season pink tennis balls at the supermarket. For salads or other fresh uses, try grape or cherry tomatoes — they're usually tastier.

Creamy Carrot Soup

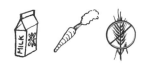

Just looking at this soup makes you feel healthy. Eating it is even better.

1 tbsp.	30 mL	butter, olive oil or vegetable oil
1		medium onion, chopped
1 lb.	500 g	carrots, diced (about 6 medium)
2 cups	500 mL	vegetable stock, homemade or store-bought (canned or from bouillon cubes or powder)
2 tbsp.	30 mL	uncooked white rice
1 tsp.	5 mL	salt
¼ tsp.	1 mL	black pepper
½ tsp.	2 mL	crumbled dried thyme
1		bay leaf
1½ cups	375 mL	milk, regular or non-dairy
1 tbsp.	15 mL	chives, chopped, if desired (but pretty)

In a large saucepan or Dutch oven, heat the butter or oil over medium heat. Add the onion and cook, stirring, for about 5 minutes, until softened.

Add the carrots, stock, rice, salt, pepper, thyme and bay leaf. Bring to a boil, and then cover the pot, reduce the heat to low and let simmer, stirring once in a while, for about 20 minutes, until carrots and rice are tender.

Fish out the bay leaf and discard. Remove the pot from the heat and let cool for about 10 minutes.

With an immersion blender (right in the pot) or in a regular blender, blend the soup until it's completely smooth. You may need to do this in two or three separate batches if using a regular blender. Return the soup to the pot if using a regular blender.

Stir in the milk and heat over medium heat until the soup is hot but not boiling.

Serve soup sprinkled with chopped chives, if you're using them.

Makes 4 servings.

Old-Fashioned Potato Soup

Here's a wonderfully comforting soup that can be made, start to finish, in just over 30 minutes. Perfect for a gloomy fall day when everything seems to be going wrong, it can also be safely (and happily) consumed on a good day.

2 tbsp.	30 mL	butter, olive oil or vegetable oil
2		medium potatoes, peeled and diced
2		medium onions, chopped
2		stalks celery, chopped
2		cloves garlic, minced or pressed
1½ cups	375 mL	vegetable stock, homemade or store-bought (canned or from bouillon cubes or powder)
1 tsp.	5 mL	salt
¼ tsp.	1 mL	black pepper
1½ cups	375 mL	milk, regular or non-dairy
		chopped chives or paprika, for garnish

Heat the butter or oil in a large saucepan or Dutch oven over medium heat. Add the potatoes, onions, celery and garlic and cook, stirring, for 6 to 8 minutes, until the onions are softened.

Add the vegetable stock, salt and pepper and bring to a boil, and then reduce the heat to medium-low, cover and simmer for 20 to 25 minutes, until the potatoes are completely falling-apart tender.

Let cool for 5 to 10 minutes.

With a potato masher (or a fork), mash the soup in the pot until there are no big lumps left.

Pour about half of the mashed soup into the container of a blender or food processor. Add the milk and blend until completely smooth.

Return the blended mixture to the mashed mixture in the saucepan, and stir to combine. This will give you a semi-smooth soup, with just enough texture to make it interesting. If you want a completely smooth soup, blend the entire soup until pureed (you may have to do this in two or three batches).

Taste and adjust the seasoning, if desired, and then place over medium heat and heat through without boiling.

Sprinkle each serving, if you like, with chopped chives or a dash of paprika for extra cheeriness.

Makes 4 to 5 servings.

Silken Cauliflower Soup

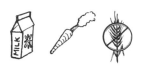

It seems almost, well, disrespectful to throw something as beautiful as a cauliflower in the blender. You'll get over it once you taste this delicious soup.

1		small cauliflower, trimmed and broken into chunks
1		medium carrot, sliced
3 cups	750 mL	vegetable stock, homemade or store-bought (canned or from bouillon cubes or powder)
⅓ cup	75 mL	uncooked white rice
2 cups	500 mL	milk, regular or non-dairy
1 tbsp.	15 mL	lemon juice
½ tsp.	2 mL	salt
¼ tsp.	1 mL	cayenne pepper
¼ tsp.	1 mL	nutmeg
		sour cream or yogurt, if desired (for garnish)

In a large pot or Dutch oven, combine the cauliflower, carrot, vegetable stock and rice. Place over medium-high heat and bring to a boil.

Reduce the heat to medium-low, cover and let cook, stirring occasionally, for about 30 minutes, until the rice is soft and the carrot and cauliflower are tender when poked with a fork.

Remove from the heat and stir in the milk.

With an immersion blender (working right in the pot) or in a regular blender or food processor, puree the soup until completely smooth. If using a regular blender or a food processor, you'll have to do this in two or three batches — it's quite a lot of soup. If using a regular blender or a food processor, return the blended soup to the pot.

Stir in the lemon juice, salt, cayenne and nutmeg.

Place over medium heat and cook until just warmed through, without letting it boil.

Serve hot or chilled, with a dollop of sour cream or yogurt on each serving.

Makes about 6 servings.

Mushroom Barley Soup

It's a dark and stormy night, but inside the kitchen you're warm and cozy because you're about to have a delicious bowl of this very comfy soup.

3 tbsp.	45 mL	butter, olive oil or vegetable oil
2		medium onions, chopped
2		medium carrots, chopped
2		cloves garlic, minced or pressed
1		stalk celery, chopped
1 lb.	500 g	mushrooms, sliced (about 5 cups/1.25 L)
3 quarts	3 L	vegetable stock, homemade or store-bought (canned or from bouillon cubes or powder)
1 cup	250 mL	pearl barley
1 tsp.	5 mL	crumbled dried thyme
1 tsp.	5 mL	salt
¼ tsp.	1 mL	black pepper
2 tbsp.	30 mL	fresh parsley, chopped

In a large pot or Dutch oven, heat the butter or oil over medium heat. Add the onions, carrots, garlic and celery and cook, stirring, for about 10 minutes, until the onions are softened.

Add the sliced mushrooms and cook for another 5 to 8 minutes, stirring often, until the mushrooms have released their juices and the liquid is beginning to evaporate.

Add the vegetable stock, barley, thyme, salt and pepper and bring to a boil over medium-high heat.

Cover the pot with a lid, reduce the heat to medium-low and let the soup cook, stirring occasionally, for 45 minutes to 1 hour, until the barley is tender. If the soup becomes too thick before the barley is cooked you may add more liquid (stock or water).

Stir in the chopped parsley and simmer for 10 to 15 minutes before serving.

Makes 8 to 10 servings.

Phenomenal Minestrone Soup

A chunky soup that's full of all kinds of good things and substantial enough to be a meal in itself. If you grate your own Parmesan cheese, save the rinds (in the freezer, if necessary) and toss them into this soup. They're an amazing flavor-booster.

2 tbsp.	30 mL	olive oil or vegetable oil
2		medium onions, chopped
4		cloves garlic, minced or pressed
4 cups	1 L	water
2		medium carrots, sliced
2		stalks celery, sliced
1 (28 oz)	1 (796 mL)	can diced tomatoes (or 3 cups/750 mL chopped fresh tomatoes)
3 (3 inch)	3 (8 cm)	chunks Parmesan cheese *rind*, or as much as you have (optional)
1 tsp.	5 mL	salt
¼ tsp.	2 mL	black pepper
1 cup	250 ml	green beans, cut into 1 inch (2 cm) pieces
½ cup	125 mL	uncooked smallish pasta, such as elbows or shells
1		medium zucchini, diced
3 cups	750 mL	spinach, roughly chopped (about ½ [10 oz/284 g] bag)
1 (19 oz)	1 (540 mL)	can white or red kidney beans, drained (2 cups/500 mL cooked dried beans)

Heat the oil in a large pot or Dutch oven over medium-high heat. Add the onion and garlic and cook, stirring occasionally, for about 5 minutes, until the onion begins to soften.

Add the water, carrots, celery, tomatoes, cheese rinds, salt and pepper. Bring to a boil, then reduce the heat to low, cover and simmer for 30 to 40 minutes, stirring occasionally.

Add the green beans and pasta and let cook for 10 minutes.

Add the zucchini, spinach and kidney beans and cook for another 10 to 15 minutes.

Fish out the cheese rinds (discard them, they've done their job) and serve the soup with additional grated Parmesan cheese to sprinkle on top.

Makes 6 to 8 servings.

Curried Butternut Squash Soup

Here's a fantastic soup: fragrant with curry and very cheerfully orange. Perfect for a crisp fall day.

2 tbsp.	30 mL	butter, olive oil or vegetable oil
1		medium onion, chopped
1 tbsp.	15 mL	curry powder
4 cups	1 L	butternut squash, peeled and cubed
2		medium potatoes, peeled and cubed
4 cups	1 L	vegetable stock, homemade or store-bought (canned or from bouillon cubes or powder)
½ cup	125 mL	milk, regular or non-dairy
1 tsp.	5 mL	salt
¼ tsp.	1 mL	black pepper

In a large pot or Dutch oven, heat the butter or oil over medium heat. Add the onion and curry powder and cook, stirring, for about 5 minutes, until the onion is softened.

Add the squash and potatoes and continue to sauté, stirring, for 1 or 2 minutes.

Pour in the stock and let it come to a boil.

Reduce the heat to low, cover the pot and let simmer for about 30 minutes, until the squash and potatoes are very soft. Let cool for a few minutes.

With a hand-held blender, working right in the pot, or in a regular blender or food processor, puree the soup until very smooth. (You may need to do this in two or three batches if working in a regular blender or a food processor). If using a regular blender or a food processor, return the soup to the pot.

Stir in the milk, salt and pepper and heat the soup until it steaming but not boiling.

Makes 4 or 5 servings.

Corn Chowder

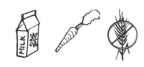

If you're using fresh corn on the cob to make this soup, you can dial up the corniness factor by simmering the stripped cobs in the vegetable stock for 10 minutes or so before using. Remove the cobs, of course, before adding the stock to the soup.

2 tbsp.	30 mL	butter, olive oil or vegetable oil
2		medium leeks or onions, trimmed and chopped
2		medium potatoes, peeled and cut into ½ inch (1 cm) cubes
4 cups	1 L	vegetable stock, homemade or store-bought (canned or from bouillon cubes or powder)
2 cups	500 mL	milk, regular or non-dairy
1 tsp.	5 mL	salt
¼ tsp.	1 mL	black pepper
4 cups	1 L	corn kernels (frozen or cut from 5 or 6 cobs)
2 tbsp.	30 mL	fresh parsley, chopped

Heat the butter or oil in a large pot or Dutch oven over medium heat. Add the leeks and cook, stirring frequently, for 5 to 7 minutes, until softened.

Add the cubed potatoes, stock, milk, salt and pepper. Bring to a boil, and then reduce the heat to medium low and let simmer for 10 to 15 minutes, until the potatoes are almost done.

Stir in the corn kernels and cook for 10 more minutes, until the corn is tender and the potatoes are very soft.

Remove about 2 cups (500 mL) of the soup and put into the container of a blender or food processor and blend until smooth.

Return the pureed portion to the pot, stir in the chopped parsley and heat through.

Makes 4 to 6 servings.

Black Bean Soup

A classic soup with a Mexican twist. Serve it with an assortment of toppings and some fresh tortillas for a full meal. Since this soup is made with dried black beans, you'll have to plan ahead if you want to make it. Worth it, though.

2 cups	500 mL	dry black beans
8 cups	2 L	water
2 tbsp.	30 mL	olive oil or vegetable oil
2		medium onions, chopped
4		cloves garlic, minced
2 tsp.	10 mL	ground cumin
1 (28 oz.)	1 (796 mL)	can diced tomatoes (or 3 cups/750 mL chopped fresh tomatoes)
1 tsp.	5 mL	crumbled dried oregano
2 tsp.	10 mL	salt
		cilantro, chopped, for serving
		cooked rice, for serving
		onion, chopped, for serving
		avocado, diced, for serving
		jalapeño pepper, chopped, for serving
		shredded cheese, for serving

Pick over the dried black beans and discard any pebbles, dirt or anything else that doesn't look like a bean. Place the beans in a large pot or Dutch oven and rinse them well in several changes of cold water. Add enough water to cover the beans by at least 2 inches (5 cm) and let them soak using either the Long Soak Method or Quick Soak Method (see page 51).

Drain and rinse the beans.

Add the 8 cups (2 L) water to the beans in the pot and bring it to a boil over medium heat.

When the beans come to a boil, reduce the heat to low and cover the pot. Let cook, stirring once in a while, for about 1 hour, until the beans are tender. For mysterious reasons, some beans will take longer to cook than others — check frequently to see how they're doing.

While the beans are cooking, heat the oil in a medium skillet over medium heat. Add the onions and cook, stirring, for about 5 minutes, until softened.

Add the garlic and cumin and continue to cook, stirring constantly, for 1 minute. Remove the pot from heat.

Once the beans are tender, add the sautéed onion mixture, the tomatoes and the oregano. Bring the mixture back to a boil over medium heat, and then reduce the heat to low and let cook for about 1 hour, partially covered (leave the cover slightly open to allow steam to escape), stirring occasionally.

Add the salt and continue to cook for another 30 minutes.

Remove 1 cup (250 mL) of the soup and put it in a blender or food processor. Blend until smooth and stir it back into the pot.

Serve the soup with an assortment of add-ins: cilantro, cooked rice, chopped onion, diced avocado, chopped jalapeño, shredded cheese or whatever else seems right.

Makes 6 to 8 servings.

Cooking Dried Beans: The Essential Guide

Yes, canned beans are quick and convenient and admittedly pretty decent. But as a vegetarian, you will eventually have to learn how to cook dried beans. It's inevitable.

Before you do anything else, place your dried beans in a bowl or strainer and pick through them to remove any pebbles or alien bits that may have gotten mixed in. Rinse well in several changes of cold water, and then place them in a large pot and add enough water to cover the beans by at least 2 inches (5 cm).

Next comes the soak. Dried beans should be soaked in water before cooking; it allows them to rehydrate, soften and will help them cook more evenly. There are two ways to do this: the Long Soak Method and the Quick Soak Method. Either method will work, so do what's most convenient for you.

Long Soak Method: Simply let the beans soak for at least 12 hours or overnight at room temperature or in the refrigerator. Drain, discarding the soaking water, then give them a quick rinse and proceed with your recipe.

Quick Soak Method: Place the pot with the beans and water on the stove over high heat. Bring to a boil, uncovered, and boil for 5 minutes. Turn off the heat, cover the pot and let the beans soak in the hot water for 1 hour. Drain, discarding the soaking water, rinse with fresh water and proceed with your recipe.

To cook: Add enough fresh water to the soaked beans to cover the beans by at least 1 inch (2 cm). Add a peeled whole onion, a couple of whole garlic cloves, maybe a slice of ginger and bring to a boil over medium heat. Don't add salt at this point (it can toughen the skins and prevent the beans from softening). Reduce the heat to medium-low, cover the pot and let the beans cook until they are tender. Depending on the type of bean and how fresh they are, this can take anywhere from 30 minutes to 2 hours. Just keep testing the beans every 15 minutes or so until they're done the way you like them. Add salt to taste once the beans are tender.

Equivalents:
1 lb. (500 g) dry beans yields approximately 6 cups (1.5 L) cooked beans.
2 cups (500 mL) drained cooked beans is equal to one 19 oz. (540 mL) can.

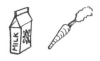

Pasta Fagioli

This is a bit of a cross between a soup and a main dish. Let's not nitpick. Whatever you want to call it, it's good, it's fast and it all gets cooked in one pot.

2 tbsp.	30 mL	olive oil
1		medium onion, chopped
2		cloves garlic, minced or pressed
1		stalk celery, chopped
4 cups	1 L	vegetable stock, homemade or store-bought (canned or from bouillon cubes or powder)
1 (28 oz.)	1 (796 mL)	can diced tomatoes (or 3 cups/750 mL chopped fresh tomatoes)
1 (19 oz.)	1 (540 mL)	can white kidney beans, drained and rinsed (or 2 cups/500 mL cooked dried beans)
1 tsp.	5 mL	salt
¼ tsp.	1 mL	black pepper
2 cups	500 mL	uncooked small pasta, such as elbows or shells
¼ cup	60 mL	fresh parsley, chopped
		grated Parmesan cheese, for sprinkling

In a large pot or Dutch oven, heat the oil over medium heat. Add the onion, garlic and celery and cook, stirring once in a while, for 4 or 5 minutes, until the vegetables are softened.

Add the stock and tomatoes and let the mixture come to a boil.

Reduce the heat to medium-low and cook, stirring once or twice, for 10 minutes.

Add the beans, salt and pepper and continue to cook for another 10 minutes.

Increase the heat to medium-high, add the pasta and cook for 8 to 10 minutes, until tender but not mushy.

Stir in the parsley for the last minute of cooking.

Serve with Parmesan cheese to sprinkle over each serving.

Makes 4 to 6 servings.

African Peanut Soup

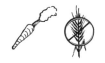

If you think that peanut butter should only ever be seen in a sandwich, think again. The peanut is actually a legume, and it probably has more in common with kidney beans than it does with a walnut or an almond. If you need more convincing, try this soup.

1 tbsp.	15 mL	olive oil or vegetable oil
2		onions, chopped
2		carrots, chopped
4 cups	1 L	vegetable stock, homemade or store-bought (canned or from bouillon cubes or powder)
¼ cup	60 mL	uncooked white rice
½ cup	125 mL	smooth peanut butter
½ tsp.	2 mL	hot pepper sauce
½ tsp.	2 mL	salt

Heat the oil in a large pot or Dutch oven over medium heat. Add the onions and carrots and cook, stirring, for 8 to 10 minutes, until the onions are soft.

Add the vegetable stock and bring to a boil.

Cover the pot, reduce the heat to low and cook, stirring occasionally, for 20 minutes.

Blend the soup until smooth using an immersion blender (working right in the pot) or in a regular blender or a food processor (in batches, if necessary). If using a regular blender or a food processor, return the blended soup to the pot.

Add the rice and cook, covered, for 15 minutes, until the rice is soft.

Stir in the peanut butter, hot pepper sauce and salt, to taste. Heat through and serve.

Makes 4 servings.

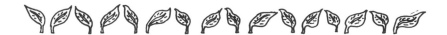

Miso Soup

This soup can be as simple as you want it to be — or as complicated. Start with a basic broth and go from there.

Broth:

4 cups	1 L	water
¼ cup	60 mL	mild miso paste (light colored)

Add-ins (choose a few):

½ cup	125 mL	diced tofu, firm or regular
2		large mushrooms, thinly sliced
1 cup	250 mL	fresh baby spinach leaves
1 cup	250 mL	cooked Japanese soba noodles (or other thin noodle)
3		green onions, sliced
1 tbsp.	15 mL	shredded dried seaweed (nori or whatever)
¼ cup	60 mL	carrot, grated

Bring the water to a boil in a medium saucepan over high heat. Remove the pan from heat and ladle about ¼ cup (60 mL) of water into a small bowl with the miso paste. Stir until the miso has mixed smoothly into the water, and then mix the diluted miso into the pot of boiled water.

Stir in whatever add-ins you like and place the pot over medium heat. Let heat through but don't bring back to a boil. Serve immediately.

Makes 3 to 4 servings.

Miso Paste

Miso is a concentrated paste made from fermented soybeans or grain and is very commonly used in Japanese cooking. It's high in protein and carbohydrates but also very salty, so it's best used sparingly — as in miso soup — or as a seasoning. Miso can be found in most Asian grocery stores or, occasionally, a supermarket with a good selection of Asian ingredients.

Chilled Zucchini Soup

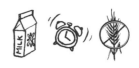

This creamy soup is absolutely delicious, almost ridiculously easy to make and the most refreshing way to start a summer meal.

4		small zucchinis, grated or chopped (about 3 cups/750 mL)
2 cups	500 mL	water
2 tbsp.	30 mL	fresh dill, chopped
1 tsp.	5 mL	salt
1 cup	250 mL	sour cream, regular or low fat
		additional sour cream and chopped dill for serving

Combine the zucchini, water, dill and salt in a large pot or Dutch oven. Place over medium-high heat and bring to a boil.

Reduce the heat to medium low and cook, stirring once or twice, for 10 minutes.

Remove from the heat, let cool to room temperature, then refrigerate until completely chilled, several hours to overnight.

Just before serving, stir the sour cream into the soup and blend until smooth and creamy, using an immersion blender right in the pot or a regular blender or food processor (in batches, if necessary).

Ladle the soup into bowls, and garnish each serving with a floating island of sour cream and, perhaps, a sprinkle of chopped dill.

Makes 4 to 6 servings.

4. Serious Salads and Dynamic Dressings

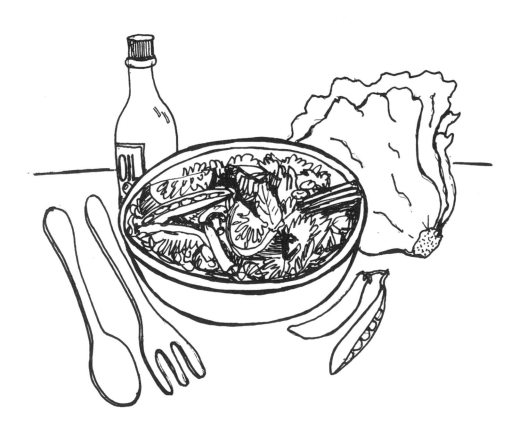

Serious Salads

Fancy French Potato Salad

Zut alors! C'est magnifique.

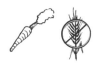

6		large new potatoes (or about 3 lbs/2.5 kg small ones)
¼ cup	60 mL	olive oil
¼ cup	60 mL	vegetable broth, homemade or store-bought (canned or from bouillon cubes or powder)
2 tbsp.	30 mL	white wine, or additional vegetable stock
2 tbsp.	30 mL	Dijon mustard
2 tbsp.	30 mL	cider vinegar or white wine vinegar
2 tbsp.	30 mL	capers, if desired (optional, but fancy and delicious)
4		green onions, chopped
1 tsp.	5 mL	salt
¼ tsp.	1 mL	black pepper

> **Mustard**
>
> A jar of Dijon mustard is an excellent thing to keep around the house. The regular yellow hot dog type mustard is fine on a hot dog but a bit harsh to use for most salad dressings or cooking purposes. Choose either a grainy or creamy Dijon — they're both great in salad dressings.

Steam or boil the whole potatoes, without peeling them, until they are tender when poked with the point of a sharp knife.

Drain thoroughly and let the potatoes cool until you can handle them easily (but don't let them cool completely).

While the potatoes are cooking and/or cooling, whisk together the olive oil, stock, wine, mustard, vinegar, capers, green onions, salt and pepper. This is your dressing. Set it aside.

Cut the potatoes into ¼-inch (0.5 cm) thick slices while they are still warm, and place them in a bowl. (Don't bother taking off the peels unless they're tough.)

Add the dressing and toss gently so that everything is evenly coated. Try not to mush up the slices.

Cover the bowl with plastic wrap and let stand at room temperature or in the refrigerator for at least 1 hour before serving. Toss again just before serving.

Makes 4 to 6 servings.

Citrus Spinach Salad

Use the freshest spinach you can find to make this salad, either tender baby spinach leaves or the regular full-grown kind will do, as long as it's crisp and fresh.

Got Strawberries?

When they're in season, substitute sliced or halved fresh strawberries for the orange in this salad and, ta da, it's Strawberry Spinach Salad. So pretty and so delicious. Sprinkle chopped or sliced almonds over top for extra crunch.

1 (10 oz.)	1 (284 g)	package fresh spinach, washed and torn into bite-sized pieces (about 6 cups/1.5 L loose leaves)
1		orange, peeled and cut into chunks
½		medium sweet onion (red onion or Vidalia are nice), thinly sliced
¼ cup	60 mL	Basic Vinaigrette Dressing (see page 76)

In a large bowl, toss together the spinach, orange chunks and onion slices.

Drizzle with Basic Vinaigrette Dressing and toss well. Gorgeous.

Makes 3 or 4 servings.

A Simple Green Salad

Begin with lettuce. Try several kinds; mix them up or buy a package of mixed baby greens.

Add some other stuff: escarole, endive, radicchio, arugula. Be brave. What could possibly go wrong? They're only leaves.

Wash and dry everything well — use a salad spinner if you have one.

Now add stuff. Tomato chunks, cucumber slices, shredded carrot, red pepper, red onion, red cabbage, radishes, whatever. Or be a purist and add nothing at all, your choice.

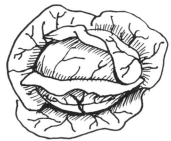

Drizzle with just enough dressing, whatever kind you like, to lightly coat the leaves, toss gently and serve immediately.

There. Simple, isn't it?

Sweet and Sour Roasted Beet Salad

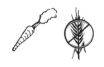

If you think you hate beets, think again. This salad may just change your mind forever.

1 lb.	500 g	fresh beets, peeled and cut into ½-inch (1 cm) chunks (about 4 or 5 medium)
1		medium red or yellow onion, cut into ½-inch (1 cm) chunks
2 tbsp.	30 mL	olive oil
1 tbsp.	15 mL	balsamic vinegar
2		cloves garlic, chopped (not pressed)
1 tsp.	5 mL	salt
¼ tsp.	1 mL	pepper
1 tbsp.	15 mL	fresh mint leaves, chopped

Preheat the oven to 400°F (200°C).

In a large, ovenproof casserole with a lid, combine the beets, onion, olive oil, balsamic vinegar, garlic, salt and pepper.

Place in the oven and bake for 45 minutes to 1 hour, until the beets are tender when poked with a fork.

Let cool slightly, then refrigerate until cold.

Just before serving, add the chopped mint and toss well. Taste and adjust seasoning if you think it needs it.

Makes 4 servings.

Balsamic Vinegar

Balsamic vinegar is wonderful in a salad — a little sweet, a little sour, very nice. Although you can pay big bucks for aged balsamic vinegar, for everyday salad dressing purposes an inexpensive bottle will do just fine. You can work your way up to the fancy stuff when you get rich.

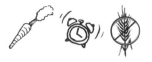

Crunchy Coleslaw

Most salads should be served as soon as they've been tossed with dressing, but this is one that breaks that rule. Since it actually gets better as it sits, make it ahead of time to let the flavors mingle and marinate.

½		small head of cabbage, finely sliced or shredded (about 8 cups/2 L)
2		green onions, chopped
1		carrot, grated
1		green sweet pepper, chopped
⅓ cup	75 mL	Basic Vinaigrette Dressing (page 76)

In a large bowl, toss together the cabbage, green onions, carrot and green pepper.

Pour the dressing over cabbage mixture and toss well.

Serve immediately, if you must, or cover tightly and refrigerate for several hours or until you're good and ready. Will keep for 3 or 4 days if refrigerated.

Makes 4 to 6 servings.

Asian Variation

Omit the Basic Vinaigrette Dressing from the recipe above and, instead, toss the salad with Sesame Ginger Dressing (see page 78) for a differently delicious twist on this old favorite.

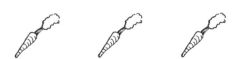

Corn and Tomato Salad

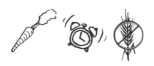

If you have a barbecue grill and a few extra minutes, try grilling the corn until lightly charred on all sides before cutting the kernels off the cob. Really, really good.

4		medium ears of corn, cooked (leftover is fine)
2		medium tomatoes, chopped
½		small red or yellow onion, chopped
2 tbsp.	30 mL	olive oil
1 tbsp.	15 mL	cider vinegar or white wine vinegar
¼ cup	60 mL	fresh basil leaves, chopped or shredded
½ tsp.	2 mL	salt
¼ tsp.	1 mL	black pepper

With a sharp knife, cut the kernels from the ears of corn and dump them into a bowl.

Add the tomatoes, onion, olive oil, vinegar, basil, salt and pepper and toss to combine thoroughly.

Serve immediately or let sit for up to an hour at room temperature.

Makes 4 servings.

Corn

Freshness counts big-time when it comes to buying corn on the cob. The moment that an ear of corn is picked from the stalk, the natural sugars that make it taste so good begin their depressing journey toward starch. Although modern hybrid corn varieties retain their sweetness longer than the older types, it's still a disappointment to bite into a gorgeous cob and find that it tastes like, well, nothing. When shopping, look for husks that are green and moist and fresh-looking silk. If you can't cook it immediately, store fresh corn in the refrigerator until ready to use.

Waldorf Salad

Crunchy, colorful and delicious — a great alternative to boring, tired winter lettuce salads.

4		medium apples
1 tbsp.	15 mL	lemon juice
1		stalk celery, diced
1 cup	250 ml	seedless grapes, halved
½ cup	125 mL	walnuts, chopped
¼ cup	60 mL	dried cranberries or raisins
½ cup	125 mL	mayonnaise
½ cup	125 mL	plain yogurt
1 tbsp.	15 mL	sugar

Core and dice the apples but don't peel them. Place in a large bowl and toss with the lemon juice.

Add the celery, grapes, walnuts and cranberries or raisins.

In a small bowl, combine the mayonnaise, yogurt and sugar.

Stir to mix, then pour over the apple mixture and toss to combine.

Cover and place in the refrigerator to chill until cold, then toss again just before serving.

Makes about 4 servings.

Warm Mushroom Salad with Goat Cheese

This is a killer first-course salad. Hardly any work, really, for something so excellent. You can make it with regular white mushrooms, but for maximum fancy-pants effect, try a mixture of whatever oddball shrooms you can get, like cremini, oyster, portobello or shiitake.

4 cups	1 L	mixed baby greens
4 tbsp.	60 mL	olive oil, divided
1		clove garlic, minced or pressed
½ lb.	250 g	fresh mushrooms, any kind or combination, sliced (about 2 cups/500 mL)
2 tbsp.	30 mL	green onions, chopped
½ tsp.	2 mL	salt
¼ tsp.	1 mL	black pepper

5 oz.	140 g	log goat cheese (with or without herbs), cut into four pieces
2 tbsp.	30 mL	balsamic vinegar (or cider vinegar with a pinch of sugar)

Preheat the oven to 375°F (190°C).

Divide the mixed baby greens equally among four plates. Set aside.

Pour 2 tbsp. (30 mL) of olive oil into a skillet and heat over medium heat. Add the garlic and cook for a minute or two, just to soften.

Dump in the mushrooms and green onions, increase the heat to high, and cook, stirring, for 2 or 3 minutes, until the mushrooms begin to release their juices.

Add the salt and pepper, stir and remove from the heat.

With a slotted spoon, remove the mushrooms from the skillet, leaving behind their juices. Divide mushrooms into four equal portions and form each portion into a little pile on cookie sheet or baking dish.

Place one piece of goat cheese on top of each pile.

Place in the oven and bake for 5 or 6 minutes, just until the cheese is heated through and begins to melt.

With a spatula, lift each mushroom and cheese pile from the baking sheet and place on top of the baby greens on each plate.

While the mushrooms are baking, you can make the dressing. Add the remaining 2 tbsp. (30 mL) of olive oil and the vinegar to the skillet with the mushroom juices.

Place over medium-high heat. Bring to a boil, scraping up any crusty bits from the bottom of the pan, and then let cook for just a minute or so.

When the salad is ready to be served, spoon the warm dressing evenly over the mushrooms, cheese and greens.

Serve immediately with good bread. Awesome.

Makes 4 servings.

Mushrooms

White button–type mushrooms are the ones you are most familiar with. They're relatively inexpensive and available everywhere, always. But don't stop there. Try portobello mushrooms: enormous, huge, walloping mushrooms that can be almost as big as a dinner plate. There is also a smaller version of this variety called crimini mushrooms. And occasionally you can find wild varieties, too, like oyster mushrooms and shiitake mushrooms. Try them all — they won't kill you, probably. No really, they won't.

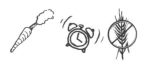

Orange and Red Onion Salad

This is perfect to serve with a spicy curry or something wildly Mexican.

4		large seedless oranges
1		small red onion
¼ cup	60 mL	cilantro, finely chopped
2 tsp.	10 mL	jalapeño pepper, finely chopped, if desired (but...)
1 tbsp.	15 mL	olive oil or vegetable oil
2 tsp.	10 mL	cider vinegar or red or white wine vinegar
½ tsp.	2 mL	salt

Peel the oranges and slice them thinly, crosswise. Place in a bowl.

Slice the red onion very thinly into rings, and then cut each ring in half and toss with the orange slices.

Add the chopped cilantro, jalapeño, oil and vinegar. Toss to combine. Sprinkle with salt and serve immediately, or let stand and serve later. Makes about 4 servings.

Bean and Barley Salad

The chewy texture of the barley helps this salad hold up when other salads have wilted and gone mushy. It's as good (maybe better) the next day.

3 cups	750 mL	water
1 cup	250 mL	pearl barley
1 (19 oz)	1 (540 mL)	can red kidney beans, drained and rinsed (or 2 cups/500 mL cooked dried beans)
1 (19 oz)	1 (540 mL)	can black beans, drained and rinsed (or 2 cups/500 mL cooked dried beans)
1 (12 oz)	1 (341 mL)	can baby corn, drained and cut into ½-inch (1 cm) pieces
1		green or red sweet pepper, chopped
1		fresh jalapeño pepper, chopped, if desired
¼ cup	60 mL	chopped green onion
½ cup	125 mL	olive oil
¼ cup	60 mL	cider vinegar or white wine vinegar
1		clove garlic, minced or pressed

½ tsp.	2 mL	ground cumin
1 tsp.	5 mL	salt
¼ tsp.	1 mL	black pepper

In a medium saucepan, combine the water and barley. Place over high heat and bring to a boil.

Reduce the heat to low, cover and let cook until all the water has been absorbed and the barley is tender, 35 to 45 minutes.

Rinse under cold running water, drain well and transfer to a large bowl.

Add the beans, corn, pepper, jalapeño and green onion.

Whisk together the oil, vinegar, garlic, cumin, salt and pepper and add to the bean mixture.

Toss well to combine, cover and place in the refrigerator to chill until ready to serve.

Serves 6 to 8.

Authentic Greek Salad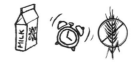

This salad is best in midsummer, made with perfectly ripe, in-season tomatoes that actually taste like, well, tomatoes. You can make a full meal out of it with the addition of some good bread and a little extra cheese. Or you can stuff it into the pocket of a pita bread and have it for lunch.

4		medium tomatoes, cut into ½-inch (1.5 cm) chunks
1		seedless English cucumber, cut into ½-inch (1.5 cm) chunks
1		red onion, coarsely chopped
⅓ cup	75 mL	Creamy Greek Dressing (see page 79)
4 oz.	125 g	feta cheese, crumbled (about 1 cup/250 mL)
½ cup	125 mL	brine-cured black olives
		salt, to taste
		black pepper, to taste

In a bowl, toss together the tomatoes, cucumber and red onion.

Add the Creamy Greek Dressing and toss to mix.

Add the feta cheese and olives and toss again.

Taste, adjust the seasoning with additional salt and pepper if you think it needs it, and serve immediately.

Makes 4 to 6 servings.

Simple Sesame Noodle Salad

If you happen to have the dressing already made, this (very simple) salad will take you no more than 10 minutes to make, start to finish.

½ lb.	250 g	Japanese soba noodles or other very thin pasta (spaghettini or angel hair)
1 tsp.	5 mL	Asian sesame oil
2		green onions, slivered
1		medium carrot, coarsely grated
¼ cup	60 mL	Sesame Ginger Dressing (see page 78)
1 tsp.	5 mL	sesame seeds, lightly toasted in a dry skillet

Bring a large pot of water to a boil over high heat. Add the noodles or other pasta and cook until tender but not mushy. (A strand should have a bit of resistance when you bite into it, but it shouldn't be chewy.)

Drain well and dump into a bowl.

Add the sesame oil and toss to coat the noodles.

Add the slivered green onions and grated carrot.

Drizzle with the Sesame Ginger Dressing and sprinkle with sesame seeds for a delicious crunch.

Makes 2 to 3 servings.

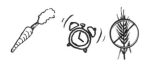

Tofu Egg Salad

Stuffed into a pita or piled onto a fresh bun with some lettuce and tomato — who knew you could make delicious egg salad without any eggs?

1 cup	250 mL	firm tofu, cut into ¼-inch (0.5 cm) cubes (about ½ [1 lb./454 g] package)
¼ tsp.	1 mL	turmeric
1		stalk celery, minced
¼		small onion, minced
¼ cup	60 mL	mayonnaise, regular or vegan (see page 81)
1 tsp.	5 mL	Dijon mustard
½ tsp.	2 mL	salt
¼ tsp.	1 mL	black pepper

Bring a medium pot of salted water to a boil over high heat. Add the diced tofu and turmeric, let the water return to a boil and cook, uncovered, for 5 minutes.

Drain thoroughly and let cool.

Place the tofu cubes in a bowl and mash them slightly with a fork.

Add the celery, onion, mayonnaise and mustard and mix well.

Sprinkle with salt and pepper and serve.

Makes 2 or 3 servings.

Variations:

- Omit the onion and add a bit of diced apple and some chopped almonds.
- Add a spoonful of pickle relish or some chopped dill pickles.
- A little hot sauce? Why not!

Give Tofu a Chance

You really have to come to terms with tofu. (If you already have, you can skip this lecture and move on to the next paragraph. If you haven't yet, then don't go anywhere.) Tofu is a perfectly harmless substance made from soybeans and can be eaten as a nutritious alternative to meat. Although occasionally ridiculed by intolerant non-vegetarians, tofu is not only a versatile and inexpensive source of protein, it's also delicious if prepared properly. As a vegetarian, you will almost certainly have to deal with it eventually. Tofu comes in many different forms and can be prepared in a gazillion different ways, quite a few of them undetectable to the naked eye. Anyone who says they don't like tofu just hasn't given it a fair shot. Keep reading.

Tofu is to beans what cheese is to milk. It's the solid protein part of the soybean, which has been prepared In such a way as to make it possible to cook In many different ways. Tofu is available in varying degrees of firmness, from really soft silken tofu (almost pudding-like) to quite hard firm tofu (with a texture like cheddar cheese). Although a particular recipe may call for a specific type of tofu, you can almost always substitute one type for another. Some people like the chewy texture of extra-firm tofu, while others prefer the soft, slippery stuff. Whatever.

Tofu is an excellent source of protein and has no cholesterol and very little fat.

Tofu itself is bland and almost tasteless, but it has a remarkable, chameleon-like ability to blend into its surroundings and absorb whatever flavors happen to be in the neighborhood. You can marinate it, if you like, or just stir-fry it with vegetables and seasonings.

Extra-firm tofu can be cut into fingers and breaded, turning it into something like chicken fingers (without the chicken). Squishy tofu can be blended into a sauce like mayonnaise or even chocolate mousse. If you freeze a block of tofu then thaw it, you can squeeze out the water and crumble it into an amazingly meat-like substance that can be added to chili, spaghetti sauce or shepherd's pie.

Now, no one is saying you should eat tofu every single day, although you could, and no one is saying you will love everything you make with it. (Even chocolate has its bad moments.) But if you're a vegetarian, tofu is certainly worth messing around with until you get it right.

All we are saying is give tofu a chance.

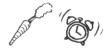

Couscous Salad

Add whatever odds and ends of vegetables you have in the house. This is a very flexible salad, and it makes an awesome lunch.

1 cup	250 mL	dry couscous
1 cup	250 mL	water
4		green onions, chopped
2		medium cucumbers, diced
2		medium green or red sweet peppers, chopped
1 (19 oz.)	1 (540 mL)	can beans, any kind (black, kidney, chickpeas), drained and rinsed (or 2 cups/500 mL cooked dried beans)
½ cup	125 mL	fresh parsley, chopped
¼ cup	60 mL	olive oil
2 tbsp.	30 mL	lemon juice
½ tsp.	2 mL	ground cumin
½ tsp.	2 mL	salt
¼ tsp.	1 mL	black pepper
		and, really, whatever else you like: canned or frozen corn, sun-dried tomatoes, olives, hot peppers, chocolate chips (just kidding)

In a medium saucepan, bring the water to a boil over high heat. Stir in the couscous, and then immediately remove the saucepan from heat and cover the pot. Let the couscous stand, covered, for 5 to 10 minutes. The couscous will absorb all the liquid.

Fluff gently with a fork to separate the granules and transfer to a large bowl.

Add the green onions, cucumbers, peppers, beans and parsley (and whatever other things you're adding to the salad). Toss gently to mix, but don't mash up the ingredients.

In a small jar, combine the oil, lemon juice, cumin, salt and pepper. Screw on the lid and shake to mix.

Pour the dressing over the couscous and toss, and then cover the bowl and chill until serving time. If the salad has absorbed all the dressing and seems a bit dry, you can toss with a bit more oil and lemon juice just before serving.

Makes 8 to 10 servings.

Thai Mango Salad

This mango salad is a version of one you may have eaten at your favorite Thai restaurant. Sometimes made with unripe green mangos, this version is made with sweet ripe ones. Addictively delicious.

2		limes, juice squeezed and zest grated
2 tbsp.	30 mL	vegetable oil
1 tbsp.	15 mL	soy sauce
1 tbsp.	15 mL	granulated sugar
½ tsp.	2 mL	crushed red pepper flakes
¼ tsp.	1 mL	salt
2		ripe mangoes, peeled and cut into strips
2		red or yellow sweet peppers, cut into strips
1		medium carrot, shredded
2		green onions, sliced
½ cup	125 ml	cilantro, chopped
6 cups	1.5 L	torn lettuce leaves (approximately)
¼ cup	60 mL	peanuts, salted or unsalted, chopped

In a small bowl, whisk together the lime juice and zest, oil, soy sauce, sugar, red pepper flakes and salt until well blended.

In a medium bowl, combine the mangoes, peppers, carrot, green onion and cilantro.

Add the dressing and toss very gently, but don't mash up the mangoes.

Line a large platter or bowl with the torn lettuce leaves.

Top with the mango mixture and sprinkle with the chopped peanuts.

To serve, make sure you scoop up some of the lettuce along with the mango mixture — delicious!

Makes 6 to 8 servings.

Chunky Pasta Salad

This veggie-packed pasta salad is a perfect picnic dish because it contains no eggs or mayo, both of which must be refrigerated for safety. For eating in the cool comfort of your own home, however, you may want to toss in a couple of hard-boiled eggs cut into wedges for a bit of extra protein.

4 cups	1 L	rotini (or other medium-sized) pasta
1 tbsp.	15 mL	olive oil or vegetable oil
2 cups	500 mL	broccoli florets
1		medium zucchini, thickly sliced
1 cup	250 mL	snow peas, halved
3		medium tomatoes, diced
¼ cup	60 mL	red or yellow onion, chopped
¼ cup	60 mL	fresh parsley, chopped
2 tbsp.	30 mL	fresh basil, chopped
⅓ cup	75 mL	Basic Vinaigrette Dressing (see page 76)
2 tbsp.	30 mL	grated Parmesan cheese
1		clove garlic, minced or pressed
		salt, to taste
		black pepper, to taste

Avoid soggy salad syndrome:

If you want to make this salad ahead of time, combine all the vegetables with the pasta but don't add the dressing. Cover and refrigerate. Toss with the dressing just before serving for a fresh sog-free pasta salad.

Bring a large pot of salted water to a boil over high heat. Add the pasta and cook until tender but not mushy.

Drain thoroughly, then rinse under cold running water and drain again. Transfer to a large bowl and toss with the oil. Let cool.

While the pasta is cooling, combine the broccoli, zucchini and snow peas in a steamer basket set over a pot of boiling water. Steam the vegetables just until the broccoli turns bright green.

Immediately remove from heat and add to the pasta in the bowl. Place in the refrigerator and chill until pasta and vegetables are cold.

When ready to serve, add the tomatoes, onion, parsley and basil to the pasta and toss to mix.

Add the Vinaigrette Dressing, Parmesan cheese and garlic and mix well. Taste and adjust the seasoning with additional salt and pepper if you think it needs it. Serve immediately.

Makes 4 to 6 servings.

Gazillion Bean Salad

Choose any combination of beans you like to make this crazily colorful salad. For maximum effect with minimum effort, use three cans of mixed beans, which is usually a combo of red and white kidney beans, chickpeas and black beans with a few others thrown in.

3 (19 oz.)	3 (540 mL)	cans any kind of beans, drained (or 6 cups/1.5 L cooked dried beans)
1		medium onion, chopped
1		medium green or red sweet pepper, chopped
1		medium tomato, diced
¼ cup	60 mL	fresh parsley or cilantro (or both), chopped
¾ cup	175 mL	Basic Vinaigrette Dressing (see page 76)
1		clove garlic, squished
2 tbsp.	30 mL	granulated sugar
		salt, to taste
		black pepper, to taste

In a large bowl, toss together the beans, onion, sweet pepper, tomato and parsley.

Add the Vinaigrette Dressing, garlic and sugar to the bean mixture and mix well. Taste and adjust the flavors with additional salt and pepper if you think it needs it.

Cover the salad and chill for at least 1 hour to allow the flavors to blend.

Toss the salad again just before serving.

Makes 6 to 8 servings.

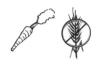

Wild and Brown Rice Salad

Serve this wonderful salad with some oven-roasted vegetables and a loaf of good bread for a great dinner.

1 cup	250 mL	uncooked brown rice
½ cup	125 mL	uncooked wild rice
2		stalks celery, thinly sliced
1		medium red onion, chopped
1		medium red or yellow sweet pepper, chopped
2 tbsp.	30 mL	fresh parsley, chopped
¼ cup	60 mL	pecans, lightly toasted, chopped
⅓ cup	75 mL	olive oil or vegetable oil
2 tbsp.	30 mL	orange juice
2 tbsp.	30 mL	lemon juice
1 tsp.	5 mL	orange zest
1 tsp.	5 mL	lemon zest
½ tsp.	2 mL	salt
¼ tsp.	1 mL	black pepper

In separate saucepans, cook the brown rice and the wild rice until tender. (See page 162 for detailed directions on cooking various kinds of rice.)

Combine the two types of rice in a large bowl and let cool to room temperature.

Once the rice has cooled, add the celery, onion, sweet pepper, parsley and pecans. Toss gently to mix — take care not to mush up the grains of rice.

In a small bowl, whisk together the oil, orange juice, lemon juice, orange and lemon zest, salt and pepper.

Pour over the rice mixture and toss gently again to mix.

Makes 4 to 6 servings.

Crunchy Carrot Salad

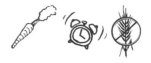

In deepest, darkest January, when even the saddest head of lettuce costs a fortune, make a colorful carrot salad instead. It's guaranteed to cheer you up.

6		medium carrots, peeled or scrubbed and shredded
2		green onions, chopped
¼ cup	60 mL	olive oil or vegetable oil
¼ cup	60 mL	lemon juice
1		clove garlic, squished
1 tsp.	5 mL	Dijon mustard
½ tsp.	2 mL	salt

Plus optional ingredients (choose one or more):

½ cup	125 mL	sunflower seed kernels
½ cup	125 mL	raisins
¼ cup	60 mL	fresh parsley, chopped
¼ cup	60 mL	cilantro, chopped
¼ tsp.	1 mL	hot pepper sauce
2 tbsp.	30 mL	fresh mint, chopped
½ tsp.	2 mL	whole or ground cumin seeds

Toss the carrots with the green onions in a large bowl.

In a small bowl, whisk together the oil, lemon juice, garlic, mustard and salt.

Drizzle the dressing over the carrot mixture and mix well.

Add any optional ingredients that happen to strike your fancy and toss again to mix.

Makes 3 or 4 servings.

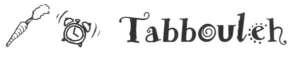

Tabbouleh

A Middle Eastern classic — light enough to serve as a side dish but hearty enough to be a main. You can toss in a can of chickpeas (drained and rinsed) to make it a bit more substantial.

1 cup	250 mL	uncooked bulgur wheat
3 cups	750 mL	boiling water
3		medium tomatoes, diced
3		green onions, chopped
½ cup	125 mL	fresh parsley, chopped
½ cup	125 mL	fresh mint, chopped (or you can omit the mint and use 1 cup/250 ml parsley)
¼ cup	60 mL	olive oil
2 tbsp.	30 mL	lemon juice
1		clove garlic (or more, or less), minced or pressed
½ tsp.	2 mL	salt
¼ tsp.	1 mL	pepper
1		cucumber, thinly sliced

Place the bulgur wheat in a large mixing bowl, add the boiling water and stir. Cover and let sit for at least 15 minutes to allow the bulgur to rehydrate. (Bulgur wheat doesn't require any further cooking when it's used in a salad; it just needs to be soaked.)

Line a strainer or a colander with a dish towel. Dump the bulgur into the towel, then lift it out and twist the whole business to wring as much water as you can out of the bulgur. The bulgur should come out fluffy and pleasantly chewy but not soggy. Transfer to a large bowl.

Add the tomatoes, green onions, parsley and mint to the bulgur in the bowl and toss to mix.

In a small bowl, whisk together the olive oil, lemon juice, garlic, salt and pepper.

Drizzle the dressing over the bulgur and vegetables and toss everything well to combine.

To serve, mound the tabbouleh up on a platter or in a bowl and decorate with cucumber slices.

Makes 4 to 6 servings.

Spicy Asian Asparagus Salad

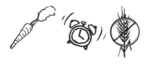

An asparagus flavor bomb — addictive with a kick.

1½ lbs.	750 g	fresh asparagus, trimmed and cut into 2-inch (5 cm) pieces
2 tbsp.	30 mL	granulated sugar
2 tbsp.	30 mL	white wine vinegar, cider vinegar or rice vinegar
2 tbsp.	30 mL	sesame oil
1 tbsp.	15 mL	Asian chili paste
1 tsp.	5 mL	salt
3 tbsp.	45 mL	vegetable oil
6		cloves garlic, cut into slivers

Place the asparagus pieces in a steamer basket over boiling water and steam for 2 to 3 minutes, just until it turns bright green. Watch carefully to avoid overcooking.

Dump the asparagus into a strainer and run cold water over it to stop it from cooking further. Let drain.

In a small bowl, combine the sugar, vinegar, sesame oil, chili paste and salt. Set aside.

In a wok or large skillet, heat the vegetable oil over high heat. Add the slivered garlic, stir for no more than 1 minute, then add the chili paste mixture and stir to mix.

Remove from heat and add the asparagus, tossing to combine well.

Cover and chill before serving — if you can wait that long.

Makes 1 serving. Just kidding. Maybe 4.

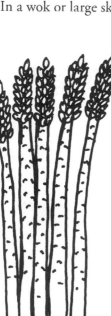

Asian Chili Paste

There are many kinds of Asian chili paste — many contain garlic, some include black beans. They all contain crushed red chiles and vegetable oil, and they are all quite spicy. For most purposes, you can use chili paste with garlic. It comes in a jar and can be found in Asian grocery stores and some large supermarkets. If you can't find it, you can substitute another hot pepper sauce in most recipes. The flavor will be different, but it will still work.

Dynamic Dressings

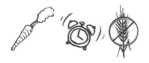 ## Basic Vinaigrette Dressing

If all else fails, make a vinaigrette. You can use it on potato salad, coleslaw, pasta salad or toss it with a bowl of mixed greens. Muck it up with garlic and herbs, add a pinch of sugar, glop in a squirt of mustard — have your way with it. It's a classic. Make the entire amount — it keeps for ages in the refrigerator and you'll always have it ready to use.

½ cup	125 mL	olive oil or vegetable oil
¼ cup	60 mL	red or white wine vinegar, cider vinegar or lemon juice
½ tsp.	2 mL	salt
¼ tsp.	1 mL	black pepper

In a small jar or bowl, combine the oil, vinegar or lemon juice, salt and pepper. Shake the jar or whisk the ingredients to mix. That's it.

Now go ahead and do something with it.

Makes ¾ cup (175 mL) dressing.

Variations on a Vinaigrette:

- Add 1 tsp. (5 mL) Dijon mustard.
- Add a minced or pressed clove of garlic.
- Sprinkle in a bit of sugar to reduce the acidity.
- Use some of that fancy walnut or hazelnut oil you got from Aunt Doris last Christmas.
- Blend in a spoonful of mayonnaise to make it creamy.
- Vary the vinegar (balsamic, anyone?).
- Add a pinch of whatever fresh or dried herbs you think might work.
- Add a squirt of ketchup (really).
- Sprinkle in some Parmesan cheese.

Sun-Dried Tomato Vinaigrette Dressing

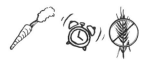

What a nifty salad dressing. Colorful and packed with flavor, it keeps almost indefinitely in the refrigerator and is perfect on a mixed green salad.

¼ cup	60 mL	sun-dried tomatoes packed in oil, chopped
¼ cup	60 mL	red or white wine vinegar or cider vinegar
2 tbsp.	30 mL	onion, minced
1 tbsp.	15 mL	water
1 or 2		cloves garlic, chopped
½ tsp.	2 mL	salt
¼ tsp.	1 mL	black pepper
1 cup	250 mL	olive oil

In the container of a blender or food processor, combine the sun-dried tomatoes, vinegar, onion, water, garlic, salt and pepper. Blend until the tomatoes are minced, and then scrape down the sides of the container and replace the lid. Turn the blender or processor back on and, with the motor running, slowly add the oil through the small opening in the lid. Blend until the dressing is thickened and creamy.

Makes about 2 cups (500 mL).

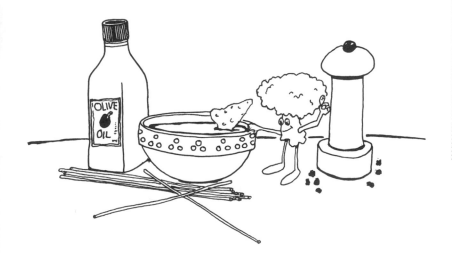

Olive Oil

A person could spend a lot of money on olive oil, but you don't have to. For salad dressings or anywhere that the flavor of the olive oil will actually matter, use extra virgin olive oil — whatever brand you can afford. The term "extra virgin" on the label means that the oil has been extracted without the use of heat or solvents. It should have a pleasant olive flavor. For cooking purposes, like for sautéeing vegetables or in spicy sauces, you can get away with ordinary olive oil (usually labeled "pure olive oil"), which is usually cheaper.

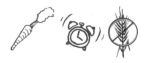

Balsamic Garlic Dressing

Here's another great dressing to keep around the house. Serve it with sturdy greens like romaine, endive, escarole, arugula or spinach. When refrigerated, olive oil has a tendency to solidify and the dressing will separate — don't be alarmed. Just let it come to room temperature before using and shake or whisk it to recombine.

1 cup	250 mL	olive oil
¼ cup	60 mL	balsamic vinegar
2		cloves garlic, chopped
1 tbsp.	15 mL	Dijon mustard
1 tsp.	5 mL	salt
1 tsp.	5 mL	black pepper

Combine all the ingredients in the container of a blender or food processor and blend until creamy. Store whatever you don't use immediately in a jar in the refrigerator.

Makes about 1½ cups (375 mL).

Sesame Ginger Dressing

This dressing is great on a salad made with Chinese cabbage (sometimes called napa cabbage), and is perfect to toss with Simple Sesame Noodle Salad (see page 66). It also makes a really nifty coleslaw (see page 60).

Sesame Oil

Sesame oil is used as a seasoning rather than a cooking oil. A little drizzle added to a stir-fry at the last minute provides a lovely sesame flavor, and it's delicious in salad dressing. There is no real substitute; simply leave it out if you don't have it. It's available in Asian grocery stores and some large supermarkets.

¼ cup	60 mL	vegetable oil
2 tbsp.	30 mL	rice vinegar
1 tbsp.	15 mL	soy sauce
1 tbsp.	15 mL	Asian sesame oil
1 tbsp.	15 mL	brown sugar
1 inch	2 cm	chunk fresh ginger root
1 tsp.	5 mL	Asian chili garlic paste (or 1 clove garlic and a pinch of crushed red pepper flakes)

Put all the ingredients into the container of a blender and blend until smooth and creamy. If you don't have a blender, whisk together the vegetable oil, vinegar, soy sauce, sesame oil and brown sugar. Mince or grate the ginger and garlic and whisk into the dressing. It won't be as creamy, but it'll still be good. (Either way, the dressing will separate if it sits for a while; just whisk or shake it together before using.)

Makes ½ cup (125 mL).

Creamy Greek Dressing

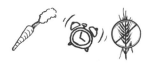

This is great to use on any green salad but is especially excellent on an Authentic Greek Salad, with tomatoes, cucumbers and feta cheese (see page 65). Keep any leftover dressing refrigerated, but let it come to room temperature before using.

⅓ cup	75 mL	lemon juice
2 tsp.	10 mL	crumbled dried oregano
1½ tsp.	7 mL	salt
1½ tsp.	7 mL	granulated sugar
½ tsp.	2 mL	black pepper
6		cloves garlic (yes, really)
1½ cups	375 mL	olive oil

Put the lemon juice, oregano, salt, sugar, pepper and garlic cloves into the container of a blender or food processor. Blend until everything is pulverized. Scrape down the sides then replace the lid. Now turn the machine back on and add the oil in a thin stream, pouring it in through the small opening in the lid while the motor is running. Blend until the dressing is thickened and creamy.

Makes about 2 cups (500 mL).

Garlic

Garlic has long been known to possess medicinal properties. It has been used to ward off disease and vampires (very useful). Serious garlic devotees will even wear a string of garlic around their necks for personal protection. How can you not love something like that? A clove of garlic is an individual section; a head of garlic is the whole thing. When shopping for garlic, look for the largest heads of garlic you can find, ones with big, firm cloves and papery white or reddish skin.

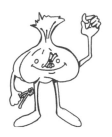

To peel a clove of garlic quickly and easily, place the clove on a flat surface, like a cutting board or table. With the side of a wide-bladed knife, whack the garlic firmly. It will get lightly crushed, and the skin will come right off.

Blue Cheese Dressing

This dressing can also double as a dip for fresh vegetables. Vary the proportion of yogurt to mayonnaise to suit your taste and the consistency you prefer.

1 cup	250 mL	plain yogurt
1 cup	250 mL	blue cheese, crumbled
½ cup	125 mL	mayonnaise
¼ cup	60 mL	green onion, including the green part, finely chopped
½ tsp.	2 mL	salt
¼ tsp.	1 mL	black pepper

Combine all the ingredients in a bowl and mix well. (For a smooth dressing, you can blend the mixture in a blender or food processor instead.)

Serve over a salad of sturdy greens or use as a dip for veggie sticks. Refrigerate any leftovers.

Makes about 2 cups (500 mL).

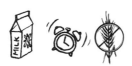

Yogurt Tahini Dressing

Drizzle over a salad of cucumbers and tomatoes or crunchy romaine or spoon into a stuffed pita sandwich. You can also use it as a dip for fresh vegetables.

1 cup	250 mL	plain yogurt
½ cup	125 mL	tahini
1		clove garlic, minced or pressed
2 tbsp.	30 mL	lemon juice
2 tbsp.	30 mL	parsley, finely chopped
1 tbsp.	15 mL	green onion, finely chopped
½ tsp.	2 mL	salt

In a blender or food processor, combine all the ingredients and blend until smooth. (You can also whisk the ingredients together in a bowl, if you prefer.)

Serve immediately or refrigerate. It will thicken in the refrigerator, making it less runny so you can use it as a dip with veggies.

Makes about 1¾ cups (425 mL).

Vegan Mayonnaise

Looks like mayo, tastes like mayo, but it's not *technically* mayo because there's no egg in it. However, if you're a vegan, that's a good thing! Use it anywhere you'd use regular mayonnaise. It will keep for about a week in the refrigerator.

1 cup	250 mL	regular (not firm) tofu (about ½ [1 lb./454 g] package)
1		clove garlic
2 tsp.	10 mL	cider vinegar
1 tsp.	5 mL	Dijon mustard
½ tsp.	2 mL	salt
¼ cup	60 mL	olive oil or vegetable oil

In the container of a blender, combine the tofu, garlic, vinegar, mustard and salt. Blend until smooth.

Turn off the blender and scrape down the sides.

With the blender running, slowly pour the oil in through the small opening in the lid, blending until the mixture is very smooth and creamy. You may have to scrape down the sides once or twice to make sure everything blends evenly.

Use immediately or spoon into a jar and refrigerate until you need it. Vegan Mayo will keep for 1 to 2 weeks if refrigerated.

Makes about 1½ cups (375 mL).

5. Exceptional Eggs and Perfect Pancakes

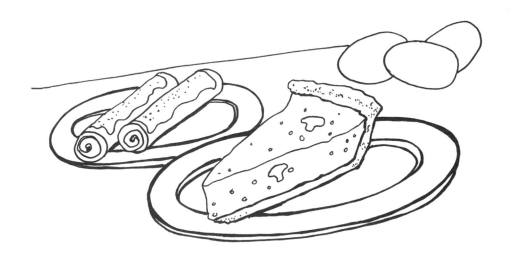

Exceptional eggs

Eggs 101

If you're a vegetarian who includes eggs in your diet, you're in luck. Eggs are just about the easiest thing to cook — quick, cheap, nutritious. Here are the three most basic ways to prepare this miracle food.

A Plain Boiled Egg

Place as many eggs as you want in a saucepan, and add enough cold water to cover the eggs by about ½ inch (1 cm).

Place the pan over medium-high heat, and as soon as the water reaches a boil, remove the pan from the burner and cover it with a lid. Begin timing:

- 1 minute for a very runny egg
- 2 minutes for a soft-boiled egg
- 4 minutes for a soft-boiled egg without any gooey spots
- 15 minutes for a hard-boiled egg

Scrambled Eggs

Crack as many eggs as you want into a bowl, and for every two eggs add 1 tbsp. (15 mL) of milk. Beat with a fork until evenly yellow.

Melt a little butter, oil or margarine in a skillet over medium-low heat. (For every every two eggs you'll need about 2 tsp./10 mL of butter or oil.)

Pour the beaten eggs into the pan and, stirring constantly, cook the eggs until they're scrambled to your taste. Some people like them softly cooked, and others like them firmly set. Suit yourself.

A Perfect Fried Egg

Melt 1 tbsp. (15 mL) butter, oil or margarine in a small skillet (non-stick, if you have it) over medium heat. Heat until the butter gets foamy, allow the foam to subside and then carefully crack the egg (or eggs) into the pan, taking great pains not to break the yolk. Lower the heat to low and let the egg cook, bubbling and spattering, until it is lightly browned on the bottom (peek underneath to check). You now have a sunnyside-up egg. If you want it over easy, *very, very* carefully flip the egg over with a spatula and let it cook for about 30 seconds, just until the top is set. Slide out onto a plate and eat.

Fabulous Frenchified Omelet

An omelet can be breakfast, lunch or dinner. It can be filled with any number of things — or with nothing at all. It's a great way to turn a couple of eggs into a dish worthy of Julia Child.

Omelet Filling Inspiration

- Diced cooked potato sautéed with onion.
- Shredded cheese — Swiss, cheddar, Asiago, whatever you have.
- Spaghetti sauce and mozzarella.
- Sautéed spinach with feta or goat cheese.
- Sautéed mushrooms with onions and garlic.
- Bean sprouts stir-fried with green onions and soy sauce.
- Ratatouille (see page 180).
- Sautéed peppers with onions and tomatoes.
- Diced apples sautéed in butter with cinnamon and sugar.

3		eggs
1 tbsp.	15 mL	water
1 tbsp.	15 mL	butter
½ tsp.	2 mL	salt
		black pepper, to taste
		omelet fillings of your choice (see sidebar for ideas)

In a small bowl, beat the eggs with the water until evenly yellow.

In a 10-inch (25 cm) skillet, heat the butter over medium heat until it's foamy, but don't allow it to get brown.

Pour the eggs into the pan, reduce the heat to medium-low and let the eggs cook, undisturbed, for just 1 minute. As the omelet begins to set underneath, gently lift the edges with a spatula and allow the uncooked egg to run under the cooked part. Keep doing this until the omelet is mostly set but still moist on top.

Sprinkle the omelet with salt and pepper and spoon whatever filling you're using onto one half of the uncooked side of the omelet.

Gently fold the un-filled half over the filled half and let the omelet continue to cook for just a moment or two to melt any cheese and heat the filling.

Carefully slide the whole thing onto a plate and serve immediately. If it sticks to the pan, slide a spatula underneath to loosen it.

Done like dinner. Repeat as needed.

Makes 1 serving.

Quickie Quiche

A quiche is a slightly more formal version of a frittata: a cheesy, eggy filling baked in a pastry crust. It's another great way to transform a humble mess of odds and ends into a delicious main dish.

2 tbsp.	30 mL	olive oil or vegetable oil
1		medium onion, chopped
1½ cups	375 mL	prepared vegetables (see sidebar for suggestions)
2 cups	500 mL	shredded Swiss or cheddar cheese
3		eggs
1 cup	250 mL	plain yogurt, regular milk or non-dairy milk
½ tsp.	2 mL	salt
¼ tsp.	1 mL	black pepper
1 (9-inch)	1 (23 cm)	unbaked pie shell, homemade or store-bought

Preheat the oven to 375°F (190°C).

Heat the oil in a medium skillet over medium heat. Add the onion and cook, stirring, for 6 to 8 minutes, until tender.

Stir in whatever raw vegetables you're using and cook for a few minutes, until just tender.

Now add any cooked vegetables you're using and heat briefly, stirring just until combined with the onion mixture.

Let cool for a minute, then spread over the bottom of the pie shell. Sprinkle with the shredded cheese.

In a small bowl, beat together the eggs and the yogurt (or milk). Add the salt and pepper and pour this mixture over the vegetables and cheese.

Place the quiche in the preheated oven and bake for 35 to 40 minutes, until puffed and golden. A knife inserted into the middle of the quiche should come out clean. Let cool for a minute or two before serving.

Makes 4 to 6 servings.

Just a Few Quiche Possibilities

- Sliced cooked or raw mushrooms
- Sliced cooked or raw zucchini
- Chopped cooked spinach
- Chopped cooked green beans
- Cooked or raw broccoli florets
- Chopped cooked or raw asparagus
- Shredded carrots
- Sliced or chopped fresh tomatoes

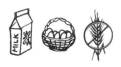

Fast Frittata

A couple of mushrooms, three stalks of asparagus, an old onion, a withered potato, can this possibly be dinner? You bet.

6		eggs, beaten
¼ cup	60 mL	olive oil or vegetable oil
1		medium onion, chopped
1½ cups	375 mL	vegetables, sliced or diced (raw mushrooms, zucchini, sweet peppers, spinach, asparagus; or cooked potatoes, green beans, corn, carrots, broccoli — use your imagination and whatever is in the fridge)
¼ cup	60 mL	grated Parmesan cheese, divided
2 tbsp.	30 mL	butter or additional olive oil
½ tsp.	2 mL	salt
¼ tsp.	1 mL	black pepper
		fresh herbs of your choice, chopped, if you have them

Crack the eggs into a large bowl and whisk them until evenly yellow. Set aside.

Heat the oil in a 10-inch (25 cm) skillet over medium heat. Add the chopped onion and cook, stirring, for about 5 minutes, until the onion is softened.

Toss in whatever raw vegetables you're using and cook for a few minutes, until they're softened.

Now add any cooked vegetables and sauté for 1 or 2 minutes, just to heat through and blend the flavors.

Transfer the vegetable mixture from the skillet to the bowl with the beaten eggs.

Add 2 tbsp. (30 mL) of the grated Parmesan cheese, the salt, pepper and whatever herbs you're using. Stir to combine.

In the same skillet you used to cook the vegetables, heat the butter or additional oil over medium heat. When the pan is hot, pour in the egg-vegetable mixture, spreading it out evenly.

Reduce the heat as low as possible and cook gently for 15 to 20 minutes, just until the eggs are set around the edges but still wobbly in the middle.

Preheat the broiler element in your oven. Adjust the top oven rack so it's as high as possible.

Sprinkle the remaining 2 tbsp. (30 mL) of Parmesan cheese over the frittata, place it under the preheated broiler and broil for 1 to 2 minutes, just until the top is set and lightly browned.

Remove the skillet from the oven, loosen the edges of the frittata with a knife and slide it out onto a plate. Or if it simply refuses to exit the pan, serve it directly from the skillet.

Cut into wedges and serve hot or let cool and serve at room temperature.

Makes 3 to 4 servings.

Broccoli Brunch Bake

This is sort of a crustless quiche, the kind of thing you can make with whatever vegetable you have around. It's delicious with broccoli, of course, but also good made with zucchini, cauliflower, leftover cooked potatoes or a mixture of vegetables, fresh or frozen.

4 cups	1 L	roughly chopped fresh broccoli (about 1 medium head)
5		eggs
2 tbsp.	30 mL	all-purpose flour
½ tsp.	2 mL	baking powder
1 cup	250 mL	cottage cheese, ricotta cheese or crumbled feta cheese
½ cup	125 mL	shredded Swiss or cheddar cheese
½ tsp.	2 mL	salt
¼ tsp.	1 mL	black pepper

Preheat the oven to 350°F (180°C). Grease an 8-inch (20 cm) square baking dish or a 9-inch (23 cm) pie pan.

Place the chopped broccoli in a steamer basket set over a pot of boiling water. Cover the pot and steam for 5 to 7 minutes, until the broccoli turns bright green and is beginning to get tender.

Transfer to the prepared baking dish, spreading it out to cover the bottom evenly.

In a medium bowl, beat the eggs with the flour and baking powder until the mixture is smooth.

Stir in the cottage, ricotta or feta cheese, mix well and pour over the broccoli in the baking dish.

Sprinkle the top with the Swiss or cheddar cheese, place in the preheated oven and bake for 25 to 30 minutes, until the center is set.

Makes about 6 servings.

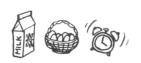

Whole-Wheat Buttermilk French Toast

Great for breakfast or brunch — awesome as a midnight snack.

2		eggs
¼ cup	60 mL	buttermilk or plain yogurt
1 tbsp.	15 mL	granulated sugar
1 tsp.	5 mL	vanilla extract
2 tbsp.	30 mL	vegetable oil
4 to 6		slices homemade-style whole-wheat bread

In a flat dish or a pie pan, beat together the eggs, buttermilk or yogurt, sugar and vanilla.

Heat the oil in a large skillet over medium heat.

Working quickly, dip the bread slices, one at a time, into the egg mixture, turning to coat both sides. Don't let the bread linger in the bowl or it will soak up too much of the egg mixture. Place as many slices in the skillet as will fit in a single layer without crowding.

Cook until golden brown then turn and cook the other side.

Remove to a plate and keep warm. Continue cooking the remaining slices of bread until they're all done. (Add a bit more oil to the pan if necessary.)

Serve hot with real honest-to-goodness maple syrup.

Makes 2 servings.

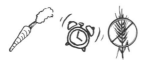

Scrambled Tofu

A vegan alternative to scrambled eggs, this is great rolled into a tortilla (with a sploosh of salsa, of course) as a breakfast burrito, or with veggies as a filling for pita pockets. It's also perfectly tasty on a plate with a toasted bagel and the Sunday crossword.

1 tbsp.	15 mL	olive oil, vegetable oil or margarine
½		medium onion, chopped
½		medium green or red sweet pepper, chopped
1 lb.	500 g	regular tofu, diced (about 2 cups/500 mL)
¼ tsp.	1 mL	turmeric
½ tsp.	2 mL	salt
¼ tsp.	1 mL	black pepper

Heat the oil or margarine in a medium skillet over medium heat. Add the onion and sweet pepper and cook, stirring occasionally, for 6 to 8 minutes, until the onion is tender.

Add the diced tofu and turmeric and cook, stirring and mashing gently, for 5 or 6 minutes, until everything is heated through and scrambled-looking.

Sprinkle with salt and pepper and serve immediately.

Makes 2 servings.

Zucchini and Basil Strata

Make this the night before you want to serve it and just pop it in the oven to bake in the morning. It's a perfect no-work dish for the morning after the night before.

6 cups	1.5 L	bread cubes (preferably stale)
2 cups	500 mL	chopped zucchini
1 cup	250 mL	shredded Swiss cheese
6		eggs
2 cups	500 mL	milk, regular or non-dairy
¼ cup	60 mL	chopped fresh basil (or 1 tbsp/15 mL dried)
¼ tsp.	1 mL	ground nutmeg
		salt, to taste
		pepper, to taste

Grease a 9 × 13–inch (23 × 33 cm) rectangular baking dish, or any deep casserole that holds 8 cups (2 L).

In the prepared baking dish, spread half the bread cubes and top with half the zucchini and half the Swiss cheese, sprinkling each layer with salt and pepper. Repeat the layers: bread, zucchini and cheese. Sprinkle the top with a bit more salt and pepper.

Beat the eggs with the milk, basil and nutmeg.

Pour the egg mixture over the bread, zucchini and cheese layers, cover with plastic wrap and refrigerate at least 2 hours or, better still, overnight.

Preheat the oven to 350°F (180°C).

Uncover the baking dish and place it in the preheated oven. Bake for 45 to 55 minutes, until slightly puffed and no longer wobbly in the middle.

Makes 6 to 8 servings.

How to Figure Out the Volume of a Baking Dish: A Ridiculously Simple Trick

Let's say you have a funny-shaped baking dish that you'd like to use. How do you know if it will hold the same amount as the boring, standard-sized dish that the recipe calls for? Easy. Fill the standard baking dish with water (measure it, if you want to be precise) then pour the water into the dish you'd like to use. If it holds the same amount of water, you're good to go.

Perfect Pancakes

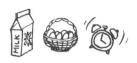

Whole-Wheat Buttermilk Pancakes

Make this breakfast classic even better by adding up to 1 cup (250 mL) of fresh or frozen blueberries to the batter. If using frozen, don't thaw them before adding.

1¼ cups	310 mL	whole-wheat flour
1 tbsp.	15 mL	granulated sugar
1 tsp.	5 mL	baking powder
½ tsp.	2 mL	baking soda
1¼ cup	310 mL	buttermilk (or see substitutes, left)
1		egg
2 tbsp.	30 mL	vegetable oil, plus more for the pan

In a large bowl, stir together the flour, sugar, baking powder and baking soda until well mixed.

Add the buttermilk, egg and oil and whisk until smooth.

Pour a small amount of oil into a large frying pan or griddle, spread it around to thinly coat the pan and place over medium heat. When a drop of water sizzles as it hits the pan, you're ready to cook.

With a spoon or ladle, pour the batter, ¼ cup (60 mL) at a time, gently spreading it out to a flat, even circle. (If the batter is too thick to pour easily, add a little more milk to thin it.)

Cook the pancake on one side until bubbles begin to appear on the top and the bottom is golden brown (peek carefully underneath to check).

With a spatula, flip the pancake over and let the other side cook until it's golden. Remove to a plate and repeat until all the batter is used. (Depending on the size of your pan, you may or may not be able to cook more than one pancake at a time.)

Makes about twelve 4-inch (10 cm) pancakes.

Buttermilk Substitutes

- Plain yogurt thinned with enough milk to make it pourable (and to equal the amount of buttermilk required in the recipe).

- For each cup (250 mL) of buttermilk required in the recipe, stir 1 tbsp. (15 mL) of vinegar into 1 cup (250 mL) of regular milk and let it sit at room temperature for 10 minutes to sour. It will curdle, but don't be alarmed. It looks yucky, but it's perfectly normal. Multiply as needed.

Featherweight Pancakes

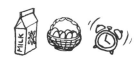

These pancakes are so light and fluffy that you may have to glue them down to your plate with maple syrup so they don't float away.

1 cup	250 mL	all-purpose white flour
2 tbsp.	30 mL	granulated sugar
2 tbsp.	30 mL	baking powder
1 cup	250 mL	milk, regular or non-dairy
1		egg
2 tbsp.	30 mL	vegetable oil, plus more for the pan

In a medium bowl, combine the flour, sugar and baking powder. (Yes, you read that right — it *is* 2 tablespoons (30 mL) of baking powder.)

In a small bowl, whisk together the milk, egg and oil. Add the milk mixture to the flour mixture and whisk until smooth.

Pour a small amount of oil into a large frying pan or griddle, spread it around to thinly coat the pan and place over medium heat. When a drop of water sizzles as it hits the pan, you're ready to cook.

With a spoon or ladle, pour the batter, ¼ cup (60 mL) at a time, gently spreading it out to a flat, even circle.

Cook the pancake on one side until bubbles begin to appear on the top and the bottom is golden brown (peek carefully underneath to check).

With a spatula, flip the pancake over and let the other side cook until it's golden. Remove to a plate and repeat until all the batter is used.

Makes about twelve 4-inch (10 cm) pancakes.

Basic Crepes

Once you get the hang of making crepes, you'll think of a million things to do with them. They're good for breakfast, lunch, dinner or dessert. See filling suggestions at right or come up with your own fabulous creations — you really can't go wrong.

1 cup	250 mL	all-purpose white flour
2		eggs
1¾ cups	425 mL	milk, regular or non-dairy
1 tsp.	5 mL	granulated sugar, if using for a sweet dish
½ tsp.	2 mL	salt, if using for a savory dish
		vegetable oil, for the pan

Put all the ingredients in a blender and blend until smooth. Pour the batter into a bowl, cover and refrigerate for at least 1 hour before using. This standing time allows the batter to thicken slightly and makes it easier to work with.

Lightly brush an 8- to 10-inch (20 to 25 cm) non-stick frying pan with vegetable oil, and place over medium heat until a drop of water sizzles as soon as it hits the pan.

Pour in about ¼ cup (60 mL) of the crepe batter, swirling the pan around to coat the bottom evenly. If necessary, use a flat spreader or knife to spread the batter out into a thin, even layer. This takes some practice, so don't feel bad if the first few crepes turn out very weird. Just eat them and say nothing.

When the top of the crepe starts to look a bit dry and the bottom is just beginning to brown (peek underneath to check), carefully flip the crepe over with a pancake turner. Cook for no more than 30 seconds — just long enough to set — then remove to a plate. (Cover and keep warm if you'll be using them right away.)

Lightly brush the pan again with oil, and repeat the process until you have used up all of the batter.

Makes 10 to 12 crepes, if all goes well.

Creative Crepe Fillings

Here are just a few suggestions for things you can roll into a crepe, both savory and sweet. But don't feel limited to these ideas. You can fill a crepe with just about anything at all, or even have them plain with a squirt of lemon juice and a sprinkle of sugar. There is simply no bad way to eat a crepe.

Savory

- Sliced mushrooms sautéed in butter, with a slosh of cream, a sprinkle of Parmesan and seasoned with parsley, salt and pepper.
- Ratatouille (see page 180).
- Sautéed sweet peppers, onions and tomatoes with shredded cheddar.
- Steamed asparagus with Pseudo-Hollandaise Sauce (see page 30).
- Steamed broccoli sprinkled with lemon juice, salt, pepper and shredded Swiss cheese.
- Use the cheese mixture from Broccoli and Cheese Stuffed Pasta Shells (see page 112), place in a baking dish, cover and bake at 350°F (180°C) for 15 to 20 minutes, until heated through.

Sweet

- Sliced apples sautéed in butter with sugar, cinnamon and lemon juice.
- Peach and Banana Flambé mixture (see page 208) served with ice cream on the side.
- Fresh strawberries, raspberries, blueberries or peaches sweetened with maple syrup and served with whipped cream.
- Apricot or strawberry jam.
- Blend some cream cheese or ricotta cheese with just enough sugar to sweeten it and add a drop of vanilla extract. Place filled crepes in a baking dish, dot with butter, cover and bake at 350°F (180°C) for 15 to 20 minutes, until heated through. Serve with fresh or defrosted frozen berries, sweetened with a bit of maple syrup or honey.
- Ice cream and chocolate sauce.

6. Marvelous Main Dishes

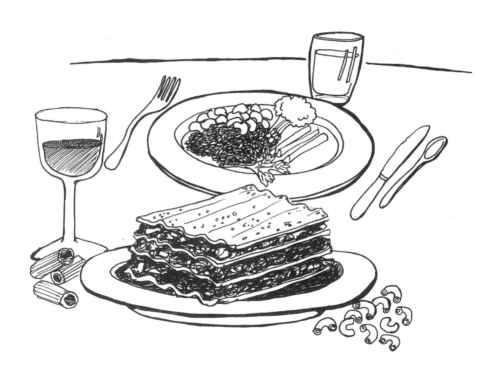

Perfect Pastas and Splendid Sauces

All-Purpose Tomato Sauce

Everyone needs a plain old reliable spaghetti sauce once in a while. This recipe makes a good-sized batch that can be tossed with pasta or used to make lasagna or pizza or in any other recipe that calls for a basic tomato pasta sauce. It also freezes well.

2 tbsp.	30 mL	olive oil or vegetable oil
1		onion, chopped
2 or 3		cloves garlic, minced or pressed
1		carrot, finely chopped
1		stalk celery, finely chopped
8 cups	2 L	chopped fresh tomatoes (about 6 lbs./3 kg. or 3 [28 oz/796 mL] cans)
2 tbsp.	30 mL	tomato paste
1 tsp.	5 mL	crumbled dried oregano
1 tsp.	5 mL	salt
½ tsp.	2 mL	black pepper
¼ cup	60 mL	fresh parsley or basil (or both!), chopped

In a large pot or Dutch oven, heat the oil over medium heat. Add the onion and garlic and cook, stirring, for 5 minutes.

Add the carrot and celery and continue to cook, stirring, for another 6 to 8 minutes, until the vegetables are beginning to soften.

Dump in the tomatoes (if you are using canned tomatoes, don't drain them), tomato paste, oregano, salt and pepper.

Bring to a boil, then reduce the heat to low and let simmer, stirring occasionally, until the sauce is thickened, about 35 to 45 minutes.

Add the parsley or basil and cook for another 5 minutes. Use immediately, spooned over freshly cooked pasta, or refrigerate or freeze to use anytime you need a plain spaghetti sauce. If you prefer a smooth texture, blend the sauce with a hand-held blender or food processor before using.

Makes about 5 cups (1.25 L), enough for 2 lbs. (1 kg) pasta or 8 to 10 servings.

Have It Your Way!

You can turn this plain spaghetti sauce into something more closely resembling, you know, meat sauce by adding some rehydrated TVP, crumbled tempeh or commercial soy hamburger substitute along with the carrot and celery at the beginning of the recipe. For a hearty, veggie-loaded sauce, add some sautéed mushrooms, zucchini or sweet peppers about halfway through the cooking time.

Perfect Pesto Sauce

Get your hands on a big bunch of fresh basil and make a batch of this wonderful pesto to use right now or stash away in the freezer. You'll be so happy you did.

½ cup	120 mL	olive oil, divided
¼ cup	60 mL	pine nuts
2 cups	500 mL	fresh basil leaves
2		cloves garlic, or more (whatever...)
½ tsp.	2 mL	salt
¾ cup	175 mL	grated Parmesan cheese, freshly grated if possible

Plenty of Other Pestobilities

- Whisk into Basic Vinaigrette Dressing (see page 76) for a pesto vinaigrette.
- Dab it onto squares of grilled polenta (see page 173) and top with a sliver of sun-dried tomato.
- Add a spoonful to Phenomenal Minestrone Soup (see page 47) before serving.
- Mix together equal amounts of pesto, yogurt and mayonnaise for a delicious dip.

Pour about 1 tbsp. (15 mL) of the olive oil into a small skillet. Add the pine nuts and place over medium-low heat, stirring constantly, until the pine nuts begin to turn golden, about 5 minutes. Warning: pine nuts can burn very quickly if you're not careful. Don't leave the pan unattended for a second while they're on the heat. (Toasting the pine nuts brings out their subtle flavor.)

Transfer the toasted pine nuts to the bowl of a food processor and add the remaining olive oil, the basil leaves, garlic and salt.

Process until almost (but not totally) smooth, scraping down the sides of the bowl a couple of times so that it blends evenly.

Add the Parmesan cheese and process just until mixed. That's it.

Makes about 2 cups (500 mL), enough to toss with 1 lb. (500 g) pasta or about 4 servings.

How to Pesto Properly

Wait! Don't just glop all that pesto over your cooked spaghetti! A proper pesto pasta should be light and creamy; it should never be gummy or overwhelming. Here's how to do it right:

Before draining your pasta, remove a cupful of pasta cooking water from the pot and set it aside. Drain the pasta in a colander and transfer it to a bowl. Add the pesto, a spoonful at a time, alternating with a drizzle of pasta-cooking water. Toss until the pasta is very lightly sauced. The pasta water will thin the sauce slightly and give the pesto a luscious, creamy consistency. Perfect. And proper.

Roasted Tomato Sauce

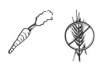

This pasta sauce is so easy it just about cooks itself. Delicious tossed with pasta, as a topping for pizza or even just spooned onto toasted baguette for a tasty bruschetta.

2 lbs.	1 kg	ripe plum tomatoes (10 to 12 medium)
4		cloves garlic, minced (don't press; you want bits, not mush)
¼ cup	60 mL	olive oil
1 tsp.	5 mL	salt
¼ tsp.	1 mL	black pepper
¼ cup	60 mL	fresh basil leaves, chopped

Preheat the oven to 425°F (220°C).

Cut the stem end off each tomato, and then cut each one lengthwise into wedges — quarters or sixths, depending on the size.

Place the tomato wedges in a large bowl and toss with the olive oil, garlic, salt and pepper.

Spread the tomatoes out on a baking sheet or shallow roasting pan large enough to hold them all in a single layer.

Place the pan in the preheated oven and bake for 35 to 40 minutes, until the tomatoes are squishy and the skins are starting to darken and wrinkle. (Don't stir or turn them at all while they're cooking.)

Remove from the oven and scoop the tomatoes into a large bowl, gently scraping the bottom of the baking pan to get all the juices and some of that nicely caramelized stuff too. Stir in the basil leaves and use immediately or refrigerate or freeze to use later.

To serve, toss with hot, cooked pasta, and pass grated Parmesan cheese at the table.

Makes about 3 cups (750 mL), enough to toss with 1 lb. (500 g) pasta or about 4 servings.

The Gluten-Free Pasta-Lover

Not such a problem anymore. Good-quality, tasty, gluten-free pasta made from rice, corn and other gluten-free grains is available just about everywhere. Pasta recipes in this section are identified as gluten-free because you can use whatever kind of pasta you prefer, regular or gluten-free. So go right ahead and indulge.

To Peel or Not to Peel...

When you're using fresh tomatoes in a recipe, a few shards of tomato peel in an otherwise delicious dish aren't really a problem. But once in a while you may feel more finicky and prefer to peel those fresh tomatoes before using them. Here's an easy way to do it:

Bring a pot of water to a boil. Stab a tomato on a fork and plunge it into the boiling water for 30 seconds. Remove it from the water and — presto! The tomato will practically peel itself. Just tug on a bit of skin and the rest of it will come off without any effort at all. Repeat until all your tomatoes are naked. Was that easy or what?

Penne with Grilled Vegetables

If you have access to a barbecue grill, this recipe may just become a summer favorite. The penne pasta is substantial enough to hold its own with the chunks of grilled vegetables, but you can use another kind of pasta (fettuccine, shells, rotini) if you prefer.

Olive-Pitting Magic Trick

Good olives generally come with pits inside them. This is annoying because most recipes ask you to take the pits out. Here's how to do it easily — no special gadget required.

Place an olive on its side on a cutting board or other flat surface. Press down firmly on the olive with the blade of a wide knife. The olive flesh will split, and you can easily remove the pit with your fingers. There. Wasn't that easy?

1½ lbs.	750 g	ripe plum tomatoes, cut in half lengthwise (about 8 medium)
2		medium onions, peeled and cut in half lengthwise
2		medium green or red sweet peppers, cut in half
1		medium zucchini, cut in half lengthwise
⅓ cup	75 mL	olive oil
¼ cup	60 mL	brine-cured black olives, pitted, chopped
¼ cup	60 mL	fresh parsley, chopped
¼ cup	60 mL	fresh basil, chopped
1 tbsp.	15 mL	capers, drained and coarsely chopped
2		cloves garlic, minced or pressed
1 tsp.	5 mL	salt
¼ tsp.	1 mL	black pepper
1 lb.	500 g	uncooked penne pasta (about 5 cups/1.25 L)
⅓ cup	75 mL	grated Parmesan cheese, plus additional for sprinkling at the table

Preheat the barbecue on high heat.

Reduce the flame on the barbecue to medium, place the tomato halves, onion halves, pepper halves and zucchini on the grill.

Cook, turning them over once, until tender and lightly charred on both sides. (Exactly how long it takes to cook each vegetable depends on the type of vegetable and the idiosyncracies of your barbecue. Just stand nearby and watch to make sure they don't burn.)

Remove the veggies from the grill as they are done and place them in a bowl. Let them stand for a few minutes to cool.

Without being obsessive about it, scrape the charred peel from the peppers and the tomatoes and chop them both up roughly. Chop the onions and zucchini also and add to the tomato mixture. Don't worry about any remaining bits of charred peel — it's all delicious.

Add the oil, olives, parsley, basil, capers, garlic, salt and pepper. (This can all be prepared several hours ahead of serving time, if you want.)

About 20 minutes before you want to serve, cook the penne in plenty of boiling salted water until tender but not mushy. Drain thoroughly, and then return the penne to the pot in which it was cooked.

Add the chopped vegetable mixture and the salt and pepper, and place over medium heat for just a minute or two, tossing until everything is heated through and combined.

Stir in the Parmesan cheese and transfer to a serving bowl.

Pass additional grated Parmesan for personal sprinkling at the table.

Makes 4 to 6 servings.

Soy Milk, Soy Cheese and Other Non-dairy Products

There are so many different types of non-dairy "milk" on supermarket shelves that it's easy to get confused. Most common are soy-based products, like soy milk, soy cheese and soy yogurt. These are made from soaked soy beans that are finely ground and strained to produce a liquid that looks pretty much like, well, cow's milk. Soy milk can be found in the refrigerated dairy case of the supermarket, just like regular milk, or in an aseptic carton (like a juice box) on the shelf, often near the canned milks. It is available in various flavors — chocolate, vanilla, natural — and can generally be used as a straight substitute for cow's milk in most recipes. You can also, of course, drink it, pour it on cereal or add it to your coffee. Soy milk is a good source of protein, and many brands are fortified with B vitamins and calcium.

Other milk substitutes are made from rice or almonds and have similar uses and nutritional benefits. Choose whichever one you like best.

Soy cheese is a rough approximation of regular dairy cheese, and it comes in different varieties, to imitate different types of cheese, such as cheddar and mozzarella. It can be used in much the same ways as regular cheese, but the results will vary with the brand; some melt better than others, and some brands have better flavor. Try several kinds until you find one that you like. It's not always going to be possible to substitute non-dairy cheese for conventional cheese in a recipe, so you'll have to experiment.

Fabulous Pasta Primavera

This stupendous pasta dish is a full-on celebration of spring. Make it with the freshest vegetables you can find and enjoy the season while it lasts.

Too Much Pasta or Rice?

Stop! Don't throw away that extra (unsauced) pasta or rice! Just pack it into containers or plastic bags and stash in the freezer. You can reheat it in a microwave or just thaw it to add to a soup or stir-fry.

1½ cups	375 mL	broccoli florets
1½ cups	375 mL	snow peas, cut in half crosswise
1 cup	250 mL	fresh or frozen peas
6		stalks asparagus, cut into 1 inch (2 cm) pieces
1		small zucchini, sliced
2 tbsp.	30 mL	olive oil
⅓ cup	75 mL	pine nuts
2		cloves garlic, minced or pressed
12		cherry tomatoes, cut in half
8		medium mushrooms, cut in quarters
1 lb.	500 g	spaghetti, linguine or fettuccine
1 cup	250 mL	half-and-half (10% cream)
¼ cup	60 mL	butter
½ cup	125 mL	Parmesan cheese, plus additional for sprinkling at the table
1 tsp.	5 mL	salt
¼ tsp.	1 mL	black pepper
⅓ cup	75 mL	fresh basil, chopped

Place the broccoli, snow peas, regular peas, asparagus and zucchini in a steamer basket set over boiling water. Steam, covered, for 2 to 3 minutes, until the colors brighten and the vegetables are tender but still crisp.

Remove from heat, transfer the vegetables to a colander and rinse under cold running water to stop them from cooking any further. Drain thoroughly and set aside.

In a large skillet, heat the olive oil over medium-low heat. Add the pine nuts and sauté for 2 to 3 minutes, until they begin to turn golden.

Add the garlic, stir for 1 minute and then increase the heat to medium high.

Add the cherry tomatoes and mushrooms and cook, stirring, for 1 minute to soften.

Now dump in all the steamed vegetables and cook, stirring, for a 1 to 2 minutes, just until everything is heated through. Remove from the heat and set aside.

Cook the pasta in a large pot of boiling salted water until tender but not mushy. Drain thoroughly and return to the pot in which it was cooked.

Add the cream, butter, Parmesan cheese, salt and pepper and cook over low heat, stirring, until the cream mixture has blended into a smooth sauce that coats the noodles.

Add the vegetable mixture and the basil and toss gently to mix.

Dump into a serving bowl and serve immediately, with additional Parmesan cheese for sprinkling at the table.

Makes 4 absolutely killer servings.

Pasta Pointers

For One Serving of Pasta

- Long pasta (like spaghetti or fettuccine) — ¾-inch (2 cm) diameter bunch.
- Medium-sized macaroni shapes (like elbows, small shells, fusilli) — 1 cup (250 mL).
- Large-sized macaroni shapes (like rotini, rigatoni, large penne) — 1½ cups (375 mL).
- Egg noodles (or other cut noodles) — 1⅔ cups (400 mL).

Unscientific Shortcut

Macaroni will approximately double in volume when cooked, so figure out what size bowl you want to end up with and fill it halfway with dry pasta. That should come out about right.

Another Unscientific Hint

A 2 lb. (900 g) package of pasta will yield about eight servings as a main dish. Use half of a package for four servings.

Vegan Alert

While most Italian-style dry pasta is made with nothing more than enriched flour and water, most fresh pasta and some varieties of dry contain some egg. And of course egg noodles will almost certainly contain egg. Get into the habit of checking the label for ingredients.

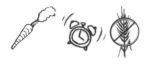

Pasta Puttanesca

A great quick, flavorful pasta sauce that can be thrown together in minutes with stuff from your pantry.

3 tbsp.	45 mL	olive oil
4		cloves garlic, minced or pressed
1 (28 oz.)	1 (796 mL)	can diced tomatoes (or about 6 large ripe tomatoes, coarsely chopped)
½ cup	125 mL	brine-cured black olives, pitted and chopped
2 tbsp.	30 mL	capers
1/3 cup	75 mL	parsley, chopped
½ tsp.	2 mL	black pepper
½ tsp.	2 mL	crushed red pepper flakes, if desired
		salt, to taste

Heat the olive oil in a large frying pan over low heat. Add the garlic and cook gently, stirring, for 2 or 3 minutes, until just starting to turn golden.

Add the tomatoes, olives and capers and continue to cook, stirring frequently, for 10 to 15 minutes, until the sauce is beginning to thicken.

Add the parsley, black pepper and red pepper flakes (if you're using them). Taste and add salt only if you think it needs it; the olives and capers are quite salty, so you may not need any additional salt.

To serve, cook the pasta until tender but firm (al dente) and drain thoroughly. Place about half the sauce in the serving bowl, add the pasta, then top with the rest of the sauce and toss well. This dish is traditionally served without cheese (but it's nobody's business what you do in the privacy of your own home).

Makes about 3 cups (750 mL), enough to toss with 1 lb. (500 g) pasta or about 4 servings.

Yes! You Can Freeze Tomatoes!

You have somehow come into a bushel of tomatoes. So you eat lots of tomato salads, and you make some spaghetti sauce. Now what will you do with the rest of them? Well, freeze them.

Nothing could possibly be easier than freezing tomatoes. Just pack them into plastic bags and throw them in the freezer. That's pretty much it. Then, when want to use some tomatoes, take out as many as you need and run them under hot water for a few seconds. The peel will practically slip right off, and you can chop the tomatoes up to use in any recipe. Don't try to use them raw, though, as they'll be mushy and watery. But cooked, they're just great.

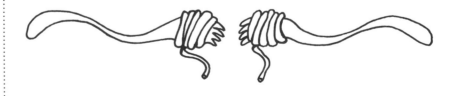

Pasta à la Caprese

This dish depends on perfectly ripe in-season tomatoes and good fresh basil. Make it on a hot day in late summer — no cooking required.

1½ lbs.	750 g	ripe plum tomatoes, roughly chopped (about 5 medium)
¼ cup	60 mL	olive oil
2		cloves garlic, minced
½		medium red or yellow sweet pepper, chopped
¼ cup	60 mL	fresh basil leaves, chopped
1 tsp.	5 mL	salt
¼ tsp.	1 mL	pepper
1 lb.	500 g	penne, shells or rotini pasta (about 5 cups/ 1.25 L)
2 cups	500 mL	mozzarella cheese, shredded or cubed (fresh water-packed mozzarella or bocconcini is fantastic in this dish, if you can get it)
		Parmesan cheese, for sprinkling at the table

In a large bowl, toss together the chopped tomatoes, oil, garlic, sweet pepper, basil, salt and pepper. Let the mixture stand, covered, at room temperature for at least 1 hour (or up to 3 hours, whatever works for you).

When you're ready to eat, cook the pasta in plenty of boiling salted water until tender but not mushy. Drain thoroughly and dump immediately into the bowl with the vegetables.

Add the mozzarella cheese and toss to combine. The heat of the pasta should soften the mozzarella and warm the tomatoes.

Serve immediately with Parmesan cheese for sprinkling at the table.

Makes 4 servings.

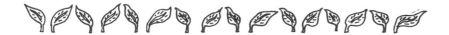

Spicy Peanut Pasta

Oddly appealing, unusually delicious, positively addictive.

Peanut sauce:

½ cup	125 mL	smooth peanut butter
½ cup	125 mL	hot water
2 tbsp.	30 mL	soy sauce
2 tbsp.	30 mL	rice vinegar or cider vinegar
2 tsp.	10 mL	sesame oil
¼ tsp.	1 mL	crushed red pepper flakes, or more, to taste
2		cloves garlic

Pasta and vegetables:

1 lb.	500 g	thin spaghetti, linguini or fresh Chinese noodles
1 tbsp.	15 mL	vegetable oil
½		medium onion, chopped
2 tsp.	10 mL	ginger root, finely grated
2 cups	500 mL	mixed stir-fry vegetables, fresh or frozen (broccoli, snow peas, sweet peppers, baby corncobs, mushrooms, whatever)
1		medium carrot, grated
2		green onions, sliced
2 tbsp.	30 mL	peanuts, salted or unsalted, chopped (whatever you have)

Fresh Ginger Root

This weird, knobby root has a wonderfully fresh, lemony flavor but with a kick. It bears no resemblance whatsoever to dried powdered ginger, so don't substitute one for the other. Refrigerated, a hunk of fresh ginger root will keep for a long time. Peel it before grating, or just ignore the peel — it's good either way.

First make the peanut sauce. In a blender or food processor, combine the peanut butter, water, soy sauce, vinegar, sesame oil, red pepper flakes and garlic. Blend until smooth. Set aside.

Cook the pasta in plenty of boiling salted water until tender but not mushy. Drain thoroughly, then rinse under cold running water drain again. Set aside.

Heat the oil in large skillet or wok over high heat. Add the onion and ginger root and stir-fry for 1 to 2 minutes.

Add the mixed vegetables and grated carrot and continue to cook, stirring and tossing constantly, just until the vegetables are tender but still crisp.

Add the cooked pasta to the pan and combine for 1 minute, then add the peanut sauce and cook just until everything is heated through.

Sprinkle with green onions and chopped peanuts and serve immediately.

Makes about 4 servings.

Bombproof Baked Macaroni Casserole

This may sound too easy to be good, but it's both: easy and good.
One pot, no pre-cooking of the pasta and totally bombproof.

1½ cups	375 mL	uncooked elbow macaroni
1 (28 oz)	1 (796 mL)	can diced tomatoes
1		small onion, chopped
1 cup	250 mL	cheddar cheese, cubed
1 cup	250 mL	water
1 tsp.	5 mL	salt
¼ tsp.	1 mL	black pepper
1 cup	250 mL	bread crumbs
1 tbsp.	15 mL	butter

Preheat the oven to 350°F (180°C). Grease a deep ovenproof casserole dish, soufflé dish or Dutch oven.

Combine the macaroni, tomatoes, onion, cheese, water, salt and pepper in the prepared baking dish. Yes, mix it all together, just like that.

Cover with the lid (or aluminum foil) and place in the preheated oven. Bake for 30 minutes.

Uncover and stir, then replace the lid and continue baking for another 30 minutes.

While the macaroni is baking, melt the butter in a small skillet over medium heat. Add the bread crumbs and cook, stirring, for 6 to 8 minutes, until the crumbs are lightly toasted.

After the casserole has baked for a total of 1 hour, remove the lid and sprinkle the buttered crumbs overtop.

Preheat the broiler element in the oven. Place the crumb-topped casserole under the broiler and broil for 3 to 5 minutes, until browned. (Watch this carefully and do not leave the room!) Let cool for just a minute or two before serving.

Makes 4 servings.

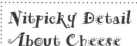

Nitpicky Detail About Cheese

Many cheeses are manufactured using an ingredient called rennet, which is an enzyme produced from the stomach of a calf (it's a by-product of veal production). If you want to avoid eating this type of product you have to learn to read cheese labels carefully. The ingredient list of vegetarian-friendly cheese will include something called vegetable rennet or microbial enzyme. If the list includes "microbial enzyme and/or rennet" or simply "rennet" you may want to choose another type of cheese.

Three-Cheese Baked Rotini

Gooey, melty cheese and plenty of it. Three different kinds, in fact! Mac and cheese just does not get much better than this.

2 cups	500 mL	grated cheddar cheese
1 cup	250 mL	grated Swiss cheese
¼ cup	60 mL	grated Parmesan cheese
8 cups	2 L	uncooked rotini pasta (about 1½ lbs./750 g)
3 tbsp.	45 mL	butter
¼ cup	60 mL	all-purpose flour
2		cloves garlic, minced or pressed
1 tbsp.	15 mL	Dijon mustard
3 cups	750 mL	milk
½ tsp.	2 mL	salt
¼ tsp.	1 mL	black pepper

Preheat the oven to 350°F (180°C). Grease a 9 x 13–inch (23 x 33 cm) rectangular baking dish.

Toss the cheeses together in a large bowl. Remove about 1 cup (250 mL) of the cheese mixture to a small bowl (this will be sprinked on top later) and set both bowls of cheese aside.

Cook the rotini in a large pot of boiling salted water until tender but not mushy. Drain in a colander, and then run cold water over it to rinse. Drain thoroughly then return it to the pot in which it was cooked.

In a medium saucepan, melt the butter over medium heat. Add the flour, garlic and mustard, and cook, stirring, for 1 to 2 minutes, until the garlic is softened.

Pour the milk in gradually while stirring or whisking to keep the mixture smooth. Cook over medium heat, stirring constantly, until the sauce thickens. Remove from the heat.

Toss the larger amount of the cheese mixture into the sauce one handful at a time, stirring as it melts. (Don't return the sauce to the heat after you've added the cheese or it may become stringy.) Add salt and pepper.

Add the cheese sauce to the cooked pasta in the pot and toss until well mixed.

Transfer to the prepared baking dish and sprinkle the remaining cheese mixture overtop.

Place in the oven and bake for 25 to 30 minutes, until it is heated through and the cheese on top is melted and bubbling.

Makes 6 to 8 servings.

Basic White Sauce

You absolutely must know how to make a basic white sauce. It can be tarted up with herbs and spices, turned into a creamy cheese sauce for pasta or served plain over steamed vegetables. Vegans can use non-dairy milk instead of regular; it will turn out just fine.

2 tbsp.	30 mL	butter, margarine or oil
2 tbsp.	30 mL	all-purpose flour
1 cup	250 mL	milk, regular or non-dairy
½ tsp.	2 mL	salt
¼ tsp.	1 mL	black pepper

Melt the butter (or margarine or oil) in a small saucepan over medium-low heat. Add the flour, and cook, stirring, for just 1 or 2 minutes.

Now slowly add the milk, increase the heat to medium and cook, stirring or whisking constantly to eliminate any lumps, until the sauce thickens and begins to simmer. Continue to cook the sauce for about 5 minutes after it reaches a simmer, stirring constantly so that it doesn't scorch and stick to the pot.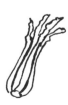

Add salt and pepper and, well, that's pretty much it.

Makes 1 cup (250 mL).

Saucy Variations:

- Add ½ cup (125 mL) shredded cheese (any kind you like) after removing the sauce from the heat. Stir until the sauce is smooth and the cheese is melted.
- Add a bit of minced onion and/or minced garlic to the butter along with the flour and cook until softened before adding the milk.
- Stir in ¼ cup (60 mL) chopped fresh parsley or basil to the sauce while it's cooking.
- Make the sauce with vegetable stock instead of milk for a lighter sauce.

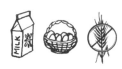

Multi-Vegetable Lasagna

This delicious lasagna uses oven-ready noodles that don't require any pre-cooking, which makes it quick to assemble (once you've got all the other components ready).

¼ cup	60 mL	olive oil or vegetable oil
1		medium onion, chopped
2		cloves garlic, minced or pressed
1 cup	250 mL	coarsely chopped mushrooms
1		small zucchini, diced
1		medium carrot, diced
1		green or red sweet pepper, chopped
4 cups	1 L	tomato pasta sauce, homemade (see page 95) or canned
1 cup	250 mL	water
2 cups	500 mL	chopped raw spinach leaves
2 cups	500 mL	ricotta cheese
2		eggs, lightly beaten
2 tbsp.	30 mL	chopped fresh parsley
½ tsp.	2 mL	salt
¼ tsp.	1 mL	black pepper
3 cups	750 mL	shredded mozzarella cheese
¼ cup	60 mL	grated Parmesan cheese
15		oven-ready (no-boil) lasagna noodles

First, make the sauce. In a large skillet or saucepan, heat the oil over medium heat. Add the onion and garlic and cook, stirring, for about 5 minutes, until softened.

Add the mushrooms, zucchini, carrot and sweet pepper and continue to cook, stirring once in a while, for 5 to 8 minutes, until the vegetables are wilted.

Now add the spaghetti sauce and water, reduce the heat to medium-low and let simmer for about 10 minutes.

Toss in the spinach and cook just until spinach collapses, a minute or two.

Taste and adjust seasoning with salt and pepper if you think it needs it; the sauce may already be sufficiently seasoned.

Now make the cheese mixture. In a bowl, mix together the ricotta, eggs, parsley, salt and pepper.

Preheat the oven to 350°F (180°C). Grease a 9 x 13–inch (23 x 33 cm) baking dish.

Now you're ready to put it all together. Spoon 1 cup (250 mL) of the sauce into the prepared baking dish and spread it out to cover the bottom.

Arrange 5 of the lasagna noodles on top of the sauce, overlapping them a bit so they cover the bottom of the pan. (You may have to break the noodles up just a bit so it all fits; that's fine, it'll be hidden once it's baked).

Cover the noodles with 2 cups (500 mL) of sauce, and then spoon on half of the ricotta cheese mixture, spreading it out in an even layer.

Sprinkle the ricotta mixture with 1 cup (250 mL) shredded mozzarella.

Repeat the layers: 5 noodles, 2 cups (500 mL) sauce, the remaining ricotta and 1 cup (250 mL) mozzarella.

Finally, top with the last 5 noodles, all the remaining sauce and the rest of the mozzarella. Sprinkle the top with Parmesan cheese.

Cover the baking dish loosely with foil, place in the preheated oven and bake for 30 minutes.

Remove the foil and continue baking for another 15 to 20 minutes, until the sauce is bubbling and a knife can easily penetrate the lasagna in the middle.

Makes about 8 servings.

Lasagna Variations:

- For a "meaty" lasagna, omit the mushrooms and zucchini in the sauce, and instead add 1½ cups (375 mL) soaked and rehydrated TVP granules, frozen and defrosted tofu (crumbled) or soy "hamburger" substitute.
- Substitute any other vegetables you like for the mushrooms, carrot, zucchini and peppers in the sauce. Just try to keep the total quantity of chopped vegetables about the same (4 cups/1 L).
- Use other cheeses instead of the mozzarella; try Swiss, Asiago, cheddar or a mixture of whatever you happen to have. It may not be traditional, but it will still be delicious.

Irresistible Mushroom Lasagna

A deliciously gooey, tomato-free lasagna layered with creamy white sauce and a pile of mushrooms. You can use whatever kind of mushrooms you like — plain white ones, brown cremini or even a mixture of different varieties.

½ cup	125 mL	butter
½ cup	125 mL	all-purpose flour
4 cups	1 L	milk
3 tsp.	15 mL	salt, divided
½ tsp.	2 mL	black pepper
1½ lbs.	750 g	fresh mushrooms, thickly sliced (8 cups/2 L)
⅓ cup	75 mL	olive oil
20		dried lasagna noodles
1 cup	250 mL	grated Parmesan cheese
1 cup	250 mL	shredded mozzarella cheese

First, make the sauce. In a large saucepan or Dutch oven, melt the butter over medium heat. Sprinkle in the flour and cook, stirring for just a minute or two, until combined.

Gradually add the milk, 1 cup (250 mL) at a time, whisking after each addition to smooth out any lumps. Continue to cook, whisking almost constantly, until the sauce thickens and just comes to a simmer, about 5 to 8 minutes.

Add 2 tsp. (10 mL) of the salt and all the pepper. Stir to mix and then remove the pan from the heat. Set aside.

Now the mushrooms. In a very large skillet or Dutch oven, heat the olive oil over medium-high heat. Add the sliced mushrooms and cook, stirring frequently, for 8 to 10 minutes, until the mushrooms soften and begin to release their juices.

Add the remaining 1 tsp. (5 mL) of salt and remove from heat. Set aside.

Now for the noodles. Bring a large pot of salted water to a boil. Add the dried lasagna noodles 3 or 4 at a time and cook for 10 minutes, until tender but not mushy or broken. As they are cooked, fish the noodles out of the pot, place in a colander and run cold water over them to rinse. Repeat until you've cooked all the noodles.

Preheat the oven to 375°F (190°C). Grease a 9 x 13–inch (23 x 33 cm) baking dish.

Now you're ready to put it all together. Spoon a small amount of sauce into the bottom of the baking dish, just enough to cover the bottom with a thin layer.

Arrange one-quarter of the noodles over the sauce, overlapping them so there are no gaps.

Spread about 1 cup (250 mL) of the sauce over the noodles and top with one-third of the mushrooms. Sprinkle with ¼ cup (50 mL) of the Parmesan.

Repeat this two more times: noodles, sauce, mushrooms, Parmesan; noodles, sauce, mushrooms, Parmesan. Finish with a top layer of noodles, the last 1 cup (250 mL) of sauce and the remaining ¼ cup (60 mL) Parmesan.

Place in the preheated oven and bake for 30 minutes.

Sprinkle the top with mozzarella cheese and bake for an additional 15 to 20 minutes, until the cheese is melted and the lasagna is bubbling around the edges.

Remove the lasagna from the oven and let it sit for about 10 minutes before serving.

Makes about 8 servings.

Lasagna Architecture Made Easy

Sauce first, then noodles, then ... cheese? Or wait — noodles, sauce, cheese, then what? Avoid confusion by drawing yourself a lasagna-building plan before you start construction. On a piece of paper, draw a simple diagram labeling each layer so that you can keep track of how many layers there should be of each component and in what order to stack them. Engineering degree not required.

Broccoli and Cheese Stuffed Pasta Shells

This is a great buffet dish. Easy to serve — even easier to eat.

24		jumbo pasta shells
1		medium bunch broccoli, coarsely chopped
1 cup	250 mL	ricotta cheese
½ cup	125 mL	shredded Swiss cheese
1		small onion, chopped
2 tbsp.	30 mL	fresh basil, chopped
½ tsp	2 mL	dried oregano, crumbled
½ tsp.	2 mL	salt
¼ tsp.	1 mL	pepper
3 cups	750 mL	tomato pasta sauce, homemade (see page 95) or canned

Cook the jumbo pasta shells in plenty of boiling salted water until they're tender but not falling apart. Drain thoroughly, rinse under cold running water and set aside.

In a steamer basket over boiling water, steam the chopped broccoli until tender but not soft, about 10 minutes. Dump into a mixing bowl and let cool for a few minutes.

Add the ricotta cheese, Swiss cheese, onion, basil, oregano, salt and pepper. Toss to combine.

Preheat the oven to 375°F (190°C). Grease a 9 x 13–inch (23 x 33 cm) rectangular baking dish.

Pour about 1 cup (250 mL) of the pasta sauce into the bottom of the prepared baking dish.

Now, working with one pasta shell at a time, spoon about 1 tbsp. (15 mL) of the cheese mixture into each shell and arrange them, open-side-up, on the sauce in the baking dish.

After the shells are all filled, pour the remaining sauce over and around the shells, and cover the pan with foil.

Bake in the preheated oven for 25 to 35 minutes, until the shells and filling are heated through and the sauce is bubbly.

Makes about 6 servings.

Stir-Fry Crazy

Basic Vegetable Stir-Fry

Here's a simple, infinitely adaptable stir-fry recipe that you can mess around with to include whatever ingredients you happen to like. The trick to a panic-free stir-fry is to have all the ingredients cut up and ready to go before you begin cooking. Once you start, it shouldn't take much more than about 10 minutes — no time to stop and slice a carrot. Pick any combination of vegetables from the list on page 114 but remember: more is not always better.

½ cup	125 mL	vegetable stock, homemade or store-bought (canned or from bouillon cubes or powder)
¼ cup	60 mL	soy sauce, regular or gluten-free
1 tbsp.	15 mL	cornstarch
2 tbsp.	30 mL	vegetable oil
1 tbsp.	15 mL	fresh ginger root, grated
2		cloves garlic, squished
10 cups	2.5 L	prepared stir-fry ingredients (see next page)

In a small bowl or measuring cup, stir together the vegetable stock, soy sauce and cornstarch. Set aside.

Heat the vegetable oil in a wok or large (12-inch/30 cm) skillet over high heat. Add the ginger and garlic and cook, stirring constantly, for 15 to 20 seconds. Don't allow the garlic to burn.

Now start tossing in the other ingredients. If you're using an onion, throw that into the wok first; it adds flavor to everything.

Next, add any firm tofu, tempeh or seitan you might be using and let it sizzle a bit, stirring constantly.

Now begin adding vegetables, starting with the dense vegetables that take longest to cook, like carrots and broccoli stems, and then add vegetables like celery, green beans, peppers and broccoli florets, followed by mushrooms and asparagus.

Finally add tender greens like spinach, bok choy, bean sprouts and shredded cabbage.

When all the vegetables are in the pan, pour in the stock mixture and, stirring constantly, cook just until the sauce thickens and becomes glossy.

Remove the pan from the heat, sprinkle with cashews, peanuts or sesame seeds, if you're using them, and serve immediately with rice or noodles.

Makes about 4 servings.

Soy Sauce

Most brands of soy sauce contain wheat as well as soy, making them unsuitable for anyone on a gluten-free diet. Gluten-free soy sauce is available, however, so you can still make a tasty stir-fry as long as you do a bit of careful label-reading when you shop.

Stir-Fry Inspirations:

- Onion, thickly sliced or cut into chunks
- Green or red sweet peppers, sliced or cut into chunks
- Carrots, sliced
- Broccoli, stems sliced and tops cut into florets
- Cauliflower, broken into florets
- Celery, sliced
- Cabbage, shredded or thinly sliced
- Bok choy, coarsely chopped
- Snow peas, trimmed
- Zucchini, sliced
- Green beans, cut into pieces
- Asparagus, cut into pieces
- Mushrooms, thickly sliced or cut into chunks
- Canned baby corncobs
- Bean sprouts
- Firm tofu or steamed tempeh or seitan, sliced or cubed
- Cashews, peanuts or sesame seeds

Sprouts

There are all sorts of sprouts out there. So how do you know what kind to buy? For cooking in a stir-fry or other Asian dish, you should look for mung bean sprouts. These are long and fleshy, usually with the actual bean hanging off the end of it. Other sprouts — alfalfa, radish, sunflower — are generally eaten raw in sandwiches and salads. Look for fresh, crisp sprouts that have been properly refrigerated, with no slimy or wilted parts — especially important if you'll be eating the sprouts uncooked. Each type has its very own distinctive taste and texture. Try them all and see which ones you like best.

And as if you didn't already have enough to do, why don't you try sprouting your own sprouts? See page 118 for details.

Spicy Garlic Tofu and Eggplant

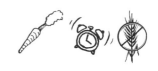

There's something about the combination of tofu and eggplant that brings out the best in both of them. Although the recipe calls for regular tofu, you can use firm tofu instead if you prefer a less squishy texture. And feel free to reduce the amount of chili paste for a milder dish — this recipe is pretty spicy.

1 lb.	500 g	regular tofu, cut into ½-inch (1 cm) cubes
1		medium regular eggplant (or 2 medium Asian eggplants), cut into ½-inch (1 cm) cubes
1 tbsp.	15 mL	soy sauce
1 tbsp.	15 mL	water
2 tsp.	10 mL	sherry or Chinese cooking wine
1 tsp.	5 mL	brown sugar
1 tsp.	5 mL	sesame oil
½ tsp.	2 mL	cornstarch
2 tbsp.	30 mL	vegetable oil
1 tbsp.	15 mL	grated fresh ginger root
2		cloves garlic, minced or pressed
2 tbsp.	30 mL	Asian chili paste
2		green onions, chopped

Place the tofu cubes in a colander or strainer set over a bowl to allow the excess water to drain out while you prepare the rest of the ingredients.

Place the eggplant cubes in a steamer basket over boiling water and steam for about 5 minutes, until soft. Remove from the heat. Set aside.

In a small bowl, stir together the soy sauce, water, sherry or wine, brown sugar, sesame oil and cornstarch. Set this aside too.

Now you're ready to start cooking. Heat the vegetable oil in a wok or large (12-inch/30 cm) skillet. Add the ginger and garlic and stir-fry for about 10 seconds.

Add the chili paste and stir for 30 seconds, until combined.

Now throw in the tofu cubes, eggplant, green onions and the soy sauce mixture. Cook, stirring constantly, until the mixture is heated through and the sauce thickens slightly.

Serve immediately with rice or noodles.

Makes 3 to 4 servings.

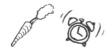

Pad Thai

It's worth looking for rice noodles to make this deliciously addictive dish. They have a wonderful chewy texture and only need to be soaked in water, not cooked, before adding to the stir-fry. If you can't find them, substitute regular fettuccine or linguine.

8 oz.	250 g	wide rice noodles (or similar quantity of fettuccine or linguine)
3 tbsp.	45 mL	lime juice
2 tbsp.	30 mL	soy sauce
2 tbsp.	30 mL	granulated sugar
1 tbsp.	15 mL	ketchup
½ tsp.	2 mL	crushed red pepper flakes
¼ cup	60 mL	vegetable oil
1 (12 oz.)	1 (350 g)	package extra-firm tofu, cut into ½-inch (1 cm) cubes
1 tbsp.	15 mL	garlic, chopped
2		eggs, beaten
2 cups	500 mL	bean sprouts, plus more to garnish
3		green onions, slivered
½ cup	125 mL	peanuts, finely chopped
¼ cup	60 mL	cilantro, chopped
		lime wedges, for serving

If using rice noodles, place the dry noodles in a large bowl, add hot tap water and let them soak for at least 30 minutes and as long as several hours. Drain and set aside. If using fettuccine or linguine, cook until tender but not mushy, rinse under cold running water and set aside.

Combine the lime juice, soy sauce, sugar, ketchup and crushed pepper flakes. Set aside.

Heat the oil in a wok or large skillet over high heat. Add the tofu and fry until golden and beginning to get crisp on all sides.

With a slotted spoon, remove the tofu to a bowl, leaving the oil behind.

Add the garlic to the pan, cook for 10 seconds and then add the eggs and cook, stirring, until scrambled.

Now add the drained noodles to the wok, mix well and pour in the soy sauce mixture.

Cook, stirring constantly, until the noodles are soft and tender, about 2 to 3 minutes. (If the noodles seem to be too dry, you can add up to ¼ cup (60 mL) of water as they cook.)

Stir in the bean sprouts and green onions, and then add the fried tofu and peanuts. Fry, tossing for 1 or 2 minutes to combine.

Taste for seasoning, adding more lime or pepper flakes if desired.

Serve sprinkled with chopped cilantro, additional bean sprouts and a wedge of lime.

Makes 3 to 4 servings.

Fried Rice with Vegetables and Un-Meat

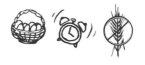

Have you ever tried seitan or tempeh? No, they're not new martial arts. They're two of the most meat-like un-meats around. Here's a great recipe to experiment with some vegetarian alternatives to chicken, beef and pork. To use tempeh or soy "stir fry strips" instead of the seitan in this recipe, see variations at side.

3 tbsp.	45 mL	vegetable oil, divided
1		egg, lightly beaten
4		green onions, sliced
1		clove garlic, squished
1		medium carrot, diced
1 cup	250 mL	peas, frozen or fresh
8 oz.	250 g	seitan, cut into 1-inch (2 cm) strips (or see sidebar)
4 cups	1 L	cooked rice (cold leftover rice is perfect)
3 tbsp.	45 mL	soy sauce

Heat 1 tbsp. (15 mL) of the oil in a large (12-inch/30 cm) skillet or wok over medium-high heat. Pour in the egg and cook, stirring constantly, until scrambled, about 2 minutes. Remove egg from the pan and set aside.

Add the remaining 2 tbsp. (30 mL) of oil to the pan and increase the heat to high. Add the green onions and garlic and stir-fry for 1 minute.

Add the carrot and peas and continue to stir-fry for 2 more minutes, until the carrot is just beginning to soften.

Add the seitan (or alternative — see sidebar) and cook for 1 more minute, stirring constantly.

Now dump in the rice, soy sauce and the scrambled egg. Stir-fry until the rice is heated through and the flavors are blended, about 2 or 3 minutes.

Serve immediately.

Makes 3 to 4 servings.

Variations on fried rice with un-meat

Instead of the seitan in the recipe above, try either:

- 8.5 oz (240 g) tempeh (approximately one package), cut into ½ inch (1 cm) cubes and steamed for 20 minutes. Proceed as for seitan.

- 8 oz. (250 g) soy "stir-fry strips" (approximately one package).

Urban Agriculture
Grow Your Own Bean Sprouts!

Just because you live in a 3rd floor walk-up apartment doesn't mean you can't grow your own food. Bean sprouts require no tractor, no giant harvesting machine, no pesticides or herbicides. All you need is some seeds, a jar, a piece of cheesecloth and a dark closet. Interested?

First, buy some mung beans at a bulk food or health food store. (Never sprout beans or seeds that are meant to be planted outdoors in a garden because they may have been treated with chemicals.) Measure about ¼ cup (60 mL) of mung beans into a 1-quart (1 L) jar. Any old kind of jar will do; it doesn't even have to have a lid. Fill the jar with cold water and cover the opening with a small square of cheesecloth or other netting fastened with a rubber band to hold it in place. Let the beans soak overnight in a dark place (like a closet). In the morning, without removing the cheesecloth, pour out the water, rinse the beans with fresh water and then drain thoroughly. Lay the jar down on its side in the dark closet and go away. Repeat the rinsing and draining two or three times a day, or whenever you think of it. The beans should just be kept moist; they shouldn't be sitting in a puddle.

After a day or two you'll begin to see small white sprouts appear. Keep rinsing and draining, and in three to five days you'll have yourself a crop ready to be harvested. The sprouts can be eaten when they're 1 to 2 inches (2.5 to 5 cm) long. Rinse well and use in any way you like.

Yee haw! Ain't farmin' fun?

Seitan

Here's a meat alternative that — surprise! — is not made from soybeans. Instead, seitan is made from wheat gluten, the protein part of wheat, and is a common meat substitute in Asian cooking. It can be cut into chunks or slices and, when marinated, has a taste and texture that comes so close to actual meat that it can make a vegetarian feel rather guilty. But don't. Seitan is perfectly innocent and totally harmless.

Although seitan may be more difficult to find than some of the other meat alternatives, you can often buy it in health food stores. It generally comes in vacuum packages, either marinated or plain. Seitan is a good source of protein, is very low in fat and has no cholesterol (of course). Since it's made from wheat, however, it's not suitable for gluten-free diets.

Because seitan is such a meat-like thing, it can be thrown, almost undetectably, into a stir-fry, stew or spaghetti sauce. For the intrepid shopper, seitan can also sometimes be found in Chinese groceries, in a canned form, usually called vegetarian duck or vegetarian pork. Very interesting stuff.

Cashew Noodle Stir-Fry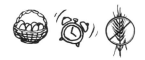

If you can find pre-cooked thin Chinese noodles (often sold in a vacuum pack in the supermarket produce section) use them in this stir-fry. They add a nice stringy, chewy texture to the dish. Otherwise use any thin cooked pasta, like spaghettini, vermicelli or capellini, instead. The chili paste makes this a spicy dish — omit it if you don't want the heat.

1 (12 oz.)	1 (350 g)	package thin pre-cooked Chinese noodles (or 8 oz./250 g spaghettini, vermicelli or capellini, cooked, drained and rinsed under cold running water)
1 tbsp.	15 mL	vegetable oil
1 cup	250 mL	cashews, whole or pieces
2		stalks celery, sliced
1		medium green or red sweet pepper, thinly sliced
1 (14 oz)	1 (398 mL)	can baby corncobs, drained and halved lengthwise
2 cups	500 mL	fresh bean sprouts
4		green onions, slivered
2 tbsp.	30 mL	soy sauce
1 tbsp.	15 mL	Asian chili paste, or less, or none

If you're using pre-cooked Chinese noodles, open the package and place them in a strainer. Pour boiling water over them and fluff them up with a fork. They're now ready to use. (If using regular pasta, just rinse under running water and set aside).

Heat the oil in a wok or large (12-inch/30 cm) skillet over high heat. Add the cashews and stir-fry for 1 minute, until they are lightly toasted. Remove from the skillet with a slotted spoon.

Add the celery, green or red pepper and baby corn and stir-fry for about 3 minutes, until the celery is tender but still crisp.

Add the bean sprouts and green onions and continue to cook for just 1 more minute, tossing constantly, until the sprouts begin to wilt.

Stir in the noodles and toss to combine.

Add the soy sauce and chili paste (if you're using it), and cook, tossing well, until everything is heated through and the flavors are combined. (If you're not using the chili paste, you may want to add another dash of soy sauce; taste it and decide for yourself.)

Sprinkle with the toasted cashews and serve immediately.

Makes 4 servings.

Chilis, Curries, Casseroles and Concoctions

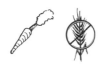 ## Chock Full of Veggies Chili

This chili is loaded with vegetables, nice and thick, and just spicy enough to make you sit up and notice.

1		large eggplant, peeled and cut into ½-inch (1 cm) cubes
2½ tsp.	12 mL	salt, divided
¼ cup	60 mL	olive oil or vegetable oil
2		onions, chopped
2		medium zucchinis, cut into ½-inch (1 cm) cubes
2		medium red or green sweet peppers, chopped
4		cloves garlic, squished
1 (28 oz.)	1 (796 mL)	can diced tomatoes (or 3 cups/750 mL chopped fresh tomatoes)
3 tbsp.	45 mL	Mexican chili powder
1 tbsp.	15 mL	ground cumin
1 tbsp.	15 mL	crumbled dried oregano
1 tsp.	5 mL	black pepper
½ tsp.	2 mL	cayenne pepper, or more or less
1 (19 oz.)	1 (540 mL)	can black, pinto or red kidney beans, drained (or 2 cups/500 mL cooked dried beans)
1½ cups	375 mL	corn kernels, frozen, canned (drained) or cut from the cob

Place the eggplant cubes in a colander set over a bowl and toss with about 2 tsp. (10 mL) of the salt. Let sit for about 1 hour to drain, then rinse and pat dry with paper towel. Salting the eggplant removes some of the liquid and helps it cook more evenly. If you are in a big hurry, you can skip this step.

Heat the oil in a large pot or Dutch oven over medium heat. Add the onions, zucchinis, sweet peppers and garlic and cook for 5 to 7 minutes, until softened.

Add the eggplant cubes and continue to cook, stirring occasionally, for 5 or 10 minutes, until the vegetables are tender.

Add the tomatoes, chili powder, cumin, oregano, pepper, cayenne and the remaining salt and bring the mixture to a boil. Lower the heat, cover the pot and cook gently, stirring once in a while, for about 15 minutes.

Add the beans and corn, and cook for another 15 minutes. Taste and adjust the seasoning if necessary.

Serve hot, sprinkled with shredded cheese if you like, and accompanied by rice or a big chunk of Jalapeño Corn Bread (see page 193).

Makes about 8 servings.

Sweet Potato and Bean Chili

This is a dirt cheap, delicious and really fast chili. You can make it with pinto beans or kidney beans for a traditional look or use black beans for a spooky Halloween effect.

2 tbsp.	30 mL	olive oil or vegetable oil
2		medium onions, chopped
2 tbsp.	30 mL	Mexican chili powder
1 tsp.	5 mL	ground cumin
2		medium sweet potatoes, peeled and cubed
1 cup	250 mL	vegetable stock, homemade or store-bought (canned or from bouillon cubes or powder)
2 (19 oz.)	2 (540 mL)	cans pinto, kidney or black beans, drained and rinsed (or 4 cups/1 L cooked dried beans)
1 (28 oz.)	1 (796 mL)	can diced tomatoes (or 4 cups/1 L chopped fresh tomatoes)
1 tsp.	5 mL	salt
1 tsp.	5 mL	crumbled dried oregano
¼ tsp.	1 mL	cayenne, or to taste
½ cup	125 mL	fresh cilantro, chopped
		shredded cheese, for serving, if desired

Heat the oil in a large saucepan or Dutch oven over medium heat. Add the onions and cook, stirring, for about 5 minutes, until onions are softened.

Add the chili powder and cumin and cook for another minute or so.

Add the sweet potatoes and vegetable stock, reduce the heat to medium-low, cover the pan and cook for 10 to 12 minutes, until the sweet potatoes are nearly tender.

Add the beans, tomatoes, salt, oregano and cayenne. Increase the heat to medium and bring to a boil.

Cover and let simmer until the sweet potatoes are completely tender, about 20 minutes.

Remove from the heat and stir in the cilantro. Serve hot with rice or corn bread and sprinkled with shredded cheese, if you like.

Makes 6 servings.

Have Your Sweet Potatoes Gone Too Far?

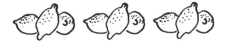

So you forgot about your sweet potatoes and they are starting to sprout in the bag. Well, all is not lost! You can turn that poor neglected vegetable into a lovely houseplant. Here's how.

Simply poke three toothpicks around the waistline of a sweet potato and suspend it vertically in a jar of water. Keep it there for a long time. As long as the potato hasn't been chemically treated to prevent sprouting, it will eventually begin to grow. First a little sprout, then a longer stem and then it turns into an attractive viney plant. Transfer it to a pot filled with potting soil once it has plenty of roots and a few leaves.

Nifty, isn't it?

Chickpea Curry

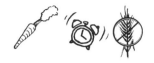

This curry is deliberately mild, but it doesn't have to be. Add a chopped fresh chile pepper or a dash of cayenne when you add the tomatoes if you want some heat.

2 tbsp.	30 mL	olive oil or vegetable oil
1		onion, chopped
1 (3-inch)	1 (7 cm)	piece cinnamon stick (or 1 pinch ground cinnamon)
2		cloves garlic, minced or pressed
1 tbsp.	15 mL	fresh ginger root, grated
1½ cups	375 mL	diced tomatoes, canned or fresh (about 3 medium tomatoes)
2 (19 oz)	2 (540 mL)	cans chickpeas, drained and liquid reserved (or 4 cups/1 L cooked dried chickpeas)
1 tsp.	5 mL	ground cumin
½ tsp.	2 mL	ground coriander
½ tsp.	2 mL	salt

Heat the oil in a large (12-inch/30 cm) skillet over medium heat. Add the onion and cinnamon and cook, stirring, for about 10 minutes, until the onion is golden.

Add the garlic and ginger and continue cooking for 1 or 2 minutes.

Dump in the tomatoes and let the mixture simmer for about 10 minutes, until the tomatoes are soft.

Stir in the drained chickpeas, cumin, coriander and salt. Bring the mixture to a simmer, and then cook, stirring occasionally, for 10 to 12 minutes. While it's cooking you may add up to 1 cup (250 mL) of reserved chickpea liquid or water to keep the mixture saucy. Remove the cinnamon stick and serve immediately with bread or rice.

Makes 4 servings.

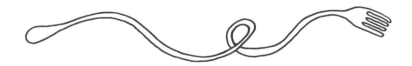

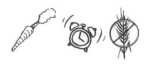

Potato and Green Pea Curry

This is the Indian equivalent of an everyday comfort dish. Good old potatoes, it seems, are good old potatoes everywhere. Leftovers, rolled in a tortilla, make a great lunch wrap.

Garam Masala

This is an Indian spice mixture that can often be found in stores that carry a good selection of spices. It usually contains cumin, coriander, cinnamon, cloves and cardamom, and it's aromatic rather than spicy. If you can't find garam masala, a reasonable substitute would be a pinch of each of the above.

2 tbsp.	30 mL	olive oil or vegetable oil
2 tsp.	10 mL	whole mustard seeds
2		onions, thickly sliced
4		cloves garlic, minced or pressed
2 tsp.	10 mL	fresh ginger root, grated
1 tsp.	5 mL	turmeric
1 tsp.	5 mL	ground cumin
1 tsp.	5 mL	garam masala (see sidebar)
½ tsp.	2 mL	salt
½ tsp.	2 mL	cayenne, or to taste (this is medium spicy)
4		medium potatoes peeled (or not) and cut into 1-inch (2 cm) cubes (about 1½ lbs./750 g)
½ cup	125 mL	water
1 cup	250 mL	frozen or fresh green peas
2 tbsp.	30 mL	fresh mint or cilantro, chopped

Heat the oil in a large skillet over medium heat. Add the mustard seeds to the oil and let them cook until they start to bounce around in the pan and pop — lots of fun to watch.

Add the onions, garlic and grated ginger. Reduce the heat to low and cook, stirring, for about 5 minutes, until the onions are softened. (Watch carefully so that the garlic and ginger don't burn.)

Add the turmeric, cumin, garam masala, salt, cayenne and potatoes. Stir around for a minute to mix and coat the potatoes with the spices.

Add the water, cover the pan and let cook, stirring once in a while, for about 15 to 20 minutes, until the potatoes are tender.

Add the peas and continue to cook for an additional 5 minutes.

Remove from heat, stir in the mint or cilantro and serve with rice or bread and some raita (see page 125) or yogurt on the side.

Makes 4 servings.

Two Refreshing Raitas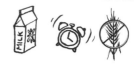

A spoonful or two of cool and creamy raita is wonderful as an accompaniment to a hot, spicy curry.

Tomato and Cucumber Raita

1½ cups	375 mL	plain yogurt
1		small tomato, finely chopped
1		small cucumber, peeled and finely chopped
1		green onion, chopped
1 tbsp.	15 mL	cilantro, chopped
½ tsp.	2 mL	salt
½ tsp.	2 mL	cumin seeds
¼ tsp.	1 mL	black pepper

Banana and Coconut Raita

1½ cups	375 mL	plain yogurt
1		ripe banana, peeled and diced
¼ cup	60 mL	grated coconut (preferably unsweetened)
1 tbsp.	15 mL	fresh mint or cilantro, chopped

Combine all the ingredients for whichever raita you're making in a bowl. Mix well and refrigerate for about 1 hour before serving to allow the flavors to blend. Makes about 2 cups (500 mL).

Leftovers Are Your Friends!

- When you're using the barbecue (if you have such a thing) grill some extra vegetables — zucchini, peppers, onions, eggplant, whatever. Marinate them in a vinaigrette dressing and refrigerate. Grilled veggies make an amazing sandwich on fresh French bread with some sliced cheese.
- Make two pizzas at once. Bake and eat one, and freeze the other. Ta da — 20 minutes and practically free!
- Turn your leftovers into TV dinners! Freeze that leftover lasagna or casserole in meal-sized portions to reheat when you're starved and in a hurry. (Do not attempt to freeze leftover salad.) For the full effect, use recycled multi-section TV dinner trays or buy sectional plates at the dollar store. Make sure you wrap trays tightly in foil or plastic wrap to prevent the food from drying out in the freezer.
- No! Stop! Don't throw out that extra rice or pasta. Just pack it into containers or plastic bags and freeze. It reheats fine in the microwave and can be thawed and added to a soup or stir-fry.

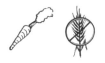

Lentil Dal

Dal is an Indian dish that's often made with lentils, but it can also be made with other types of legumes. It tends to be soupy and is usually served with rice as part of an Indian meal. You can even roll it into a warm flour tortilla for a quick meal on the run. A little spicy, in a very good way.

1 cup	250 mL	dried brown or green lentils
4 cups	1 L	water
1 tsp.	5 mL	salt
2 tbsp.	30 mL	fresh ginger root, grated
½ tsp.	2 mL	turmeric
¼ tsp.	1 mL	ground cardamom
¼ tsp.	1 mL	cayenne pepper
2 tbsp.	30 mL	vegetable oil
½ tsp.	2 mL	crushed red pepper flakes
½ tsp.	2 mL	ground cumin
2 tbsp.	30 mL	cilantro, chopped
2 tbsp.	30 mL	lemon juice

Pick over the lentils, then rinse them well and place in a medium saucepan. Add the water and salt and bring to a boil over medium heat.

Reduce the heat, cover the pot and let the lentils simmer for 45 minutes, stirring occasionally.

Add the ginger, turmeric, cardamom and cayenne and continue to simmer for another 10 to 15 minutes, until the lentils are completely soft, adding a bit more water, if necessary (the mixture should be like a thick soup).

Meanwhile, heat the oil in a small skillet over medium heat. Add the red pepper flakes and cumin and cook, stirring, for 2 or 3 minutes.

Stir this mixture into the lentils along with the chopped cilantro and lemon juice. Serve hot with rice and a refreshing raita (see page 125).

Makes 4 servings.

Thai Green Curry with Tofu and Vegetables

And by green, we certainly don't mean cool. Thai green curries can be fiery hot, but since you're doing the cooking here, you can adjust the level of heat by adding more or less of the green curry paste. Serve this veggie-packed curry over rice.

1 (14 oz.)	1 (398 mL)	can "light" coconut milk, divided
½		medium onion, chopped
2		cloves garlic, minced or pressed
1 tsp.	5 mL	fresh ginger root, grated
1 to 2 tbsp.	15 to 30 mL	Thai green curry paste (see sidebar)
½ (12 oz.)	½ (350 g)	package extra-firm tofu, cut into ½-inch (1 cm) cubes
1		medium carrot, cut into ½-inch (1 cm) cubes
1		medium zucchini, cut into ½-inch (1 cm) cubes
2 cups	500 mL	broccoli florets (save the stems for another use)
2 tbsp.	30 mL	cilantro, chopped
2 tbsp.	30 mL	fresh basil, chopped

Pour ½ cup (125 mL) of the coconut milk into a large skillet. Bring it to a boil over medium heat, and then add the onion, garlic and ginger root. Cook, stirring, for 2 minutes.

Add the green curry paste (start with the smaller amount, taste and add more if you want). Cook, stirring for 2 minutes, until the curry paste has dissolved.

Add the tofu and carrot to the pan and cook, stirring often, for 6 to 8 minutes, until the carrot is nearly tender.

Add the zucchini and broccoli and cook for about 5 minutes, just until the broccoli and zucchini are tender but still bright green.

Stir in the cilantro and basil and serve immediately with rice.

Makes 3 or 4 servings.

Thai Curry Paste

Thai curry paste is a prepared seasoning mixture for Thai curries that can be found in many Asian grocery stores and in some large supermarkets. It comes in various colors -— green, red and yellow are most common. Each type is made with a specific blend of herbs and spices and, although many Thai curry pastes are completely vegetarian, some do include shrimp or fish extract among the ingredients. You'll have to do some label-reading to make sure the brand you buy is vegetarian.

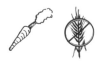

Eight-Vegetable Stew

Snuggle up to a bowl of this delicious stew on a cold winter evening. It'll make you feel all warm and cozy.

Veggie Pot Pie: What a Concept

After the stew has finished cooking, dump it into an ovenproof baking dish and top with a layer of rolled-out and cut Biscuit Mix dough (see page 194). Bake at 375°F (190°C) for about 20 minutes, until the biscuits are browned. Lovely.

¼ cup	60 mL	olive oil or vegetable oil
3		cloves garlic, minced or pressed
2 cups	500 mL	small whole mushrooms (about ½ lb./250 g)
1½ cups	375 mL	whole baby carrots (about ½ lb./250 g)
1 cup	250 mL	white wine or vegetable stock
2 cups	500 mL	vegetable stock, homemade or store-bought (canned or from bouillon cubes or powder)
2		medium potatoes, peeled and cut into ½-inch (1 cm) cubes
2 tbsp.	30 mL	tomato paste
¼ cup	60 mL	fresh parsley, chopped
1 tsp.	5 mL	salt
¼ tsp.	1 mL	black pepper
12		pearl onions, peeled (about ¼ lb./125 g)
2 cups	500 mL	broccoli florets
1		medium red sweet pepper, cut into strips
1		medium zucchini, cut into ½-inch (1 cm) chunks
1 cup	250 mL	cauliflower florets

Heat the oil in a large pot or Dutch oven over medium heat. Add the garlic, mushrooms and carrots and sauté for 2 or 3 minutes, stirring constantly.

Add the wine or stock, increase the heat to medium-high and cook, stirring, until the liquid is reduced by about half, about 5 to 7 minutes.

Add the 2 cups (500 mL) vegetable stock, potatoes, parsley, tomato paste, salt and pepper. Cover and cook, stirring frequently, for about 10 minutes, until the potatoes are almost tender.

Now toss in the pearl onions, broccoli, red pepper, zucchini and cauliflower and continue to cook, stirring once in a while, for another 5 to 7 minutes, until all the vegetables are tender.

Serve immediately with some good bread, rice or quinoa to sop up the delicious sauce.

Makes 4 servings.

Spicy Vegetable Couscous

This spicy vegetable concoction can also be served with rice, quinoa, bread or pasta if you don't happen to have any couscous in the house.

1 tbsp.	15 mL	olive oil or vegetable oil
1		medium onion, chopped
2		cloves garlic, minced or pressed
1 cup	250 mL	butternut squash, peeled and cut into ½-inch (1 cm) cubes
1 cup	250 mL	vegetable stock, homemade or store-bought (canned or from bouillon cubes or powder)
1		medium zucchini, cut into ½-inch (1 cm) cubes
1 (19 oz.)	1 (540 mL)	can chickpeas, drained (or 2 cups/500 mL cooked dried chickpeas)
½ tsp.	2 mL	ground cumin
½ tsp.	2 mL	curry powder
¼ tsp.	1 mL	crushed red pepper flakes, or more (if you dare)
1		medium tomato, cut into chunks (or ½ cup/125 mL canned diced tomato)
¼ cup	60 mL	raisins
1 tsp.	5 mL	salt
¼ tsp.	1 mL	black pepper
1 cup	250 mL	dry couscous
1 cup	250 mL	boiling water

Stop and Smell the Roses

Or, in this case, the vegetables. Take a few minutes before you begin cooking to prepare all the vegetables and arrange them (artistically) on a platter. This step may take longer than the actual cooking itself, but it cuts down on frantic last-minute chopping and gives you an opportunity to admire all the colorful vegetables before they're thrown into the pot.

In a large pot or Dutch oven, heat the oil over medium heat. Add the onion and garlic and cook until softened, about 5 minutes.

Add the butternut squash and vegetable stock, cover and let simmer until the squash is almost tender, about 15 minutes.

Add the zucchini, chickpeas, cumin, curry powder and hot pepper flakes and stir. Replace the cover and let the mixture cook for about 5 minutes.

Add the tomato, raisins, salt and pepper and cook until heated through.

While the vegetable mixture is simmering, prepare the couscous. Place the dry couscous in a bowl or saucepan. Pour the boiling water over it, stir and then cover and let sit for 10 minutes. Fluff with a fork and scoop into a serving bowl. (That's all there is to it.)

When the vegetable mixture is done, scoop the couscous into a large serving bowl and make an indentation in the middle of it, like a volcano. Spoon the vegetable mixture into the crater and serve immediately.

Makes 3 to 4 servings.

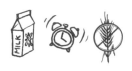

Mushroom Stroganoff with Seitan (or Not)

This meatless version of a classic dish is packed with delicious mushrooms in a creamy sauce. Elegant comfort food.

Where's the Beef? Not Here

If you can find seitan in your local health food store and you've never used it, this recipe is a perfect way to try it. Seitan (wheat gluten, not scary, see page 118) has a chewy, meaty texture that goes very nicely with the mushrooms and adds protein besides. For a gluten-free version, you can either substitute soy stir-fry strips or omit it altogether and throw in a few extra mushrooms.

1 tbsp.	15 mL	olive oil or vegetable oil
9 oz.	250 g	seitan, cut into 1/8-inch (0.25 cm) slices (see sidebar)
1 tbsp.	15 mL	butter or additional oil
1 lb.	500 g	mushrooms, cut into quarters (about 5 cups/1.25 L)
1		onion, chopped
½ cup	125 mL	white wine
1 tbsp.	15 mL	all-purpose flour
1 cup	250 mL	vegetable stock, homemade or store-bought (canned or from bouillon cubes or powder)
¼ cup	60 mL	sour cream
2 tbsp.	30 mL	fresh parsley, chopped
½ tsp.	2 mL	salt
¼ tsp.	1 mL	black pepper

Heat the oil in a large skillet over medium heat. Add the seitan slices (if you're using it) and fry them, turning the slices over as they become slightly crisp and golden. Remove from the pan, leaving as much as the oil behind as possible, and set aside.

Add the butter to the frying pan and let it melt. Dump in the mushrooms and onion and cook, stirring, over medium heat for 8 to 10 minutes, until the mushrooms have released their liquid and it has mostly cooked away.

Add the wine and cook for about 3 minutes, until it is slightly reduced.

Sprinkle the flour over the mushrooms, stir and then pour in the stock and bring the mixture to a boil.

Return the seitan slices to the pan, lower the heat and let simmer for a couple of minutes or until the sauce has thickened.

Stir in the sour cream, parsley, salt and pepper. Heat through but don't let it boil. Serve immediately with buttered noodles or plain cooked rice.

Makes 2 servings.

Cuban-Style Black Beans

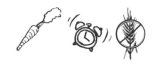

Crank up the heat and put some Cuban music on the stereo and — hey! — you're dining in Havana. Well, almost.

¼ cup	60 mL	olive oil or vegetable oil
4		cloves garlic, squished
1		medium onion, chopped
1		medium red sweet pepper, chopped
2 tsp.	10 mL	crumbled dried oregano
2 (19 oz.)	2 (540 mL)	cans black beans, drained (or 4 cups/1 L cooked dried beans)
1 cup	250 mL	vegetable stock, homemade or store-bought (canned or from bouillon cubes or powder)
2 tbsp.	30 mL	vinegar
1 tsp.	5 ml	salt
¼ tsp.	1 ml	black pepper

Heat the oil in a large saucepan or Dutch oven over medium heat. Add the garlic, onion, sweet pepper and oregano and cook, stirring, for 5 to 7 minutes, until the onions are softened.

Add about one-quarter of the beans to the pan and mash them with a fork.

Pour in the rest of the beans, the vegetable stock, vinegar, salt and pepper and let simmer for about 15 minutes, stirring once in a while. Serve immediately with plain white rice or Coconut Rice (see page 163).

Makes 4 to 6 servings.

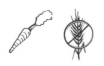

Nearly Normal Shepherd's Pie

This is so close to the meat-based original that it seems almost like cheating. But if you're a new vegetarian who's pining for old comfort foods or if you're looking for a family meal that is definitely not weird, this is absolutely perfect.

1½ cups	375 mL	TVP granules (see box, page 133)
1½ cups	375 mL	vegetable stock, homemade or store-bought (canned or from bouillon cubes or powder), heated to boiling
¼ cup	60 mL	olive oil or vegetable oil
1		onion, chopped
2		cloves garlic, squished
½ lb.	250 g	mushrooms, sliced (about 2½ cups/625 mL)
1		medium red or green sweet pepper, diced
1		medium carrot, diced
1 cup	250 mL	fresh or frozen peas or corn kernels
1 cup	250 mL	ketchup, spaghetti sauce or salsa (or a mixture)
1 tsp.	5 mL	salt
¼ tsp.	1 mL	black pepper
1 recipe		Fluffy Mashed Potatoes (see page 174) paprika, for garnish

Preheat the oven to 350°F (180°C). Lightly grease a 9-inch (23 cm) square baking dish.

In a bowl, combine the TVP granules with the hot vegetable stock and let soak while you prepare the rest of the ingredients.

Heat the oil in a large skillet over medium heat. Add the onion and garlic and cook, stirring, for 5 minutes, until the onions are softened.

Add the mushrooms, peppers and carrot and cook, stirring often, for 6 to 8 minutes, until the carrots are starting to soften.

Reduce the heat to medium low, add the soaked TVP to the skillet (all the liquid will have been absorbed by the granules) and cook, stirring occasionally to prevent sticking, for about 5 minutes.

Add the peas or corn, ketchup (or whatever sauce you're using), salt and pepper and continue cooking, stirring once in a while. If the mixture seems too dry, add up to ½ cup (125 mL) water or stock to the skillet (the mixture should be about the thickness of a hearty chili).

Transfer to the prepared baking dish and spread it out evenly.

In the meantime, make the Fluffy Mashed Potatoes (see page 174). While still warm, spread the potatoes over the mixture in the baking dish, smoothing out the surface or making ripples with a fork or decorating it in some creative way or another. Sprinkle the top with paprika.

Place in the preheated oven and bake for 35 to 40 minutes, until the top is golden and the veggie mixture underneath is hot and bubbling around the edges. Serve immediately.

Makes 4 to 6 nearly normal servings.

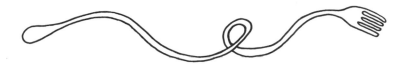

Textured Vegetable Protein (TVP)

Textured vegetable protein, also known as TVP or textured soy protein, is a protein-rich meat substitute made from soy flour. It's a dry, granular product that's great to use in chili or spaghetti sauce. TVP adds a chewy, meaty texture when rehydrated and simmered in a flavorful sauce.

TVP is about 70 percent protein, making it highly nutritious, and it retains most of the soy bean's dietary fiber. It can be found in natural or bulk food stores and may have different brand names, depending on the manufacturer. In its dry form, TVP can be stored at room temperature (like cereal), but it must be rehydrated in boiling water or vegetable stock before using.

Using TVP in place of ground beef in a portion of a recipe — chili, spaghetti sauce or shepherd's pie — makes it easy to accommodate both vegetarians and non-vegetarians without cooking two entirely separate meals.

Baked Polenta with Spinach and Cheese

Polenta is cooked cornmeal that is often served instead of pasta in an Italian meal. It can be a side dish like mashed potatoes, but sometimes polenta is baked into layered casseroles like this one.

1 recipe		Basic Oven-Baked Polenta (see page 173)
1 (10 oz.)	1 (284 g)	package fresh spinach leaves (about 6 cups/1.5 L loose leaves)
1 cup	250 mL	ricotta cheese
2 tbsp.	30 mL	fresh parsley, chopped
½ tsp.	2 mL	salt
¼ tsp.	1 mL	black pepper
2 cups	500 mL	shredded mozzarella cheese
¼ cup	60 mL	grated Parmesan cheese

Preheat the oven to 350°F (180°C). Grease a 9-inch (23 cm) square baking dish.

First prepare the Basic Oven-Baked Polenta according to the recipe on page 173. Since it takes almost 1 hour to cook, begin baking the polenta before you start to prepare the rest of the recipe. That way it will be done when you're ready for it.

While the polenta is cooking, rummage through the spinach leaves and remove any thick stems or wilted bits. Rinse well, then place the wet leaves into a large saucepan. Place over medium-high heat and cook, covered, stirring occasionally, until the spinach has completely collapsed, about 3 or 4 minutes.

Drain the spinach well and chop coarsely. Set aside.

In a small bowl, mix the ricotta cheese with the parsley, salt and pepper. Set this aside too.

When the polenta is done, and while it's still hot and soft, pour about half of it into the prepared baking dish, spreading it out in a smooth layer. Top with the chopped spinach, then the ricotta cheese mixture and sprinkle with half of the shredded mozzarella and half of the Parmesan cheese. Spoon the rest of the polenta on top, and sprinkle with the rest of the mozzarella and Parmesan cheeses.

Bake in the preheated oven for 35 to 40 minutes, or until bubbly and beginning to brown on top.

Makes 4 to 6 servings.

Incredible Onion Tart

You might not think that a tart filled with nothing but, well, onions could really be this good, but it is. Incredible, isn't it?

Crust

1 cup	250 mL	biscuit mix, homemade (see page 194) or store-bought
1/3 cup	75 mL	milk, regular or non-dairy
1 tsp.	5 mL	crumbled dried sage

Filling

¼ cup	60 mL	butter
4		medium onions, thinly sliced
1		egg
½ cup	125 mL	milk, regular or non-dairy
½ tsp.	2 mL	salt
¼ tsp.	1 mL	black pepper

Preheat the oven to 400°F (200°C).

First make the crust. In a medium bowl, stir together the biscuit mix, milk and sage.

Squish the dough into the bottom and up the sides of an 8-inch (20 cm) pie plate. Set aside.

Now the filling. Melt the butter in a large skillet over medium-low heat. Add the onions and cook, stirring occasionally, for 12 to 15 minutes, until the onions are golden.

Let cool slightly, then dump into the biscuit-lined pie plate.

In a small bowl, beat together the egg, milk, salt and pepper and pour over the onions in the pan.

Place in the preheated oven and bake for 20 to 25 minutes, until the top is lightly browned and the pie is set (a knife poked into the middle should come out clean). Serve immediately.

Makes 4 servings.

Vegetarian Moussaka

Moussaka is the perfect dish to serve when you're entertaining carnivorous friends or family. Who could care that there's no meat when they're eating something so good? Singing, dancing and plate-smashing after dinner are optional (but fun).

2		medium eggplants, sliced ½-inch (1 cm) thick (don't peel)
		salt
2 tbsp.	30 mL	olive oil, approximately (for brushing eggplant)

Vegetable sauce

2 tbsp.	30 mL	olive oil
2		medium onions, chopped
2		cloves garlic, minced or pressed
1		medium zucchini, diced
½		medium red or green sweet pepper, diced
1 tsp.	5 mL	crumbled dried oregano
½ tsp.	2 mL	salt
¼ tsp.	1 mL	cinnamon
¼ tsp.	1 mL	black pepper
2 cups	500 mL	diced tomatoes, fresh (about 4 medium) or canned
3 tbsp.	45 mL	tomato paste

Custard sauce

2 tbsp.	30 mL	butter
2 tbsp.	30 mL	flour
¾ cup	175 mL	milk
1 tsp.	5 mL	salt
¼ tsp.	1 mL	nutmeg
¼ tsp.	1 mL	black pepper
2		eggs, lightly beaten
1 cup	250 mL	ricotta cheese
1 cup	250 mL	feta cheese, crumbled

Generously sprinkle salt on both sides of the eggplant slices and stand them upright (as much as possible) in a colander over a bowl that will catch the drips. Let the eggplant stand for at least 30 minutes. (This step helps remove some of the water from the eggplant so that it cooks more evenly and may reduce any bitterness.) Rinse slices and pat dry with paper towel.

Adjust the top oven rack to 4 inches (10 cm) from the upper element and preheat the broiler. Grease a 9 x 13–inch (23 x 33 cm) baking dish.

Working in batches, brush the eggplant slices on both sides with the olive oil. Arrange on a cookie sheet in a single layer (don't crowd).

Place on the top oven rack and broil until lightly browned, turning the slices over once to brown both sides. Repeat with the remaining eggplant slices until they're all browned. Set aside.

Now make the tomato sauce. Pour the 2 tbsp. (30 mL) of olive oil into a large skillet over medium-high heat. Add the onions, garlic, zucchini and sweet pepper and cook, stirring, for 5 to 7 minutes, until the vegetables are softened.

Stir in the oregano, salt, cinnamon and pepper and cook for 1 to 2 minutes, to blend the flavors.

Add the tomatoes and tomato paste, lower the heat to medium-low and cook, stirring often, for about 10 minutes, until slightly thickened.

Finally, make the custard sauce. In a medium saucepan, melt the butter over medium heat. Sprinkle in the flour and cook, stirring, for 1 to 2 minutes, until blended.

Add the milk and cook, stirring or whisking constantly, until smooth and thickened.

Remove from the heat and whisk in the eggs, ricotta, salt, nutmeg and pepper. Set aside.

Now put it all together. Spread half of the vegetable sauce in the prepared baking dish, and top with half of the eggplant slices, arranging them so they're in a single layer.

Sprinkle with half of the feta cheese.

Repeat with the remaining tomato sauce and the rest of the eggplant.

Spread the custard sauce over the top and sprinkle with the remaining feta cheese.

At this point you may bake the moussaka immediately or cover and refrigerate up to 24 hours before baking.

When ready to bake, preheat the oven to 350°F (180°C).

Place the moussaka in the preheated oven and bake, uncovered, for 50 to 60 minutes, until the top is browned and the eggplant mixture underneath is bubbling around the edges.

Let it stand for about 15 minutes before serving.

Makes 6 to 8 servings.

Spanakopita

The phyllo crust makes this impressive-looking dish seem like a lot of work (not true). It tastes as delicious as it looks. Read the hints, below, for working with phyllo if you've never used it before.

2 (10 oz.)	2 (284 g)	packages fresh spinach (about 12 cups/3 L loose leaves)
½ cup	125 mL	butter, divided
1		medium onion, chopped
1½ cups	375 mL	feta cheese, crumbled (about ½ lb./250 g)
2 cups	500 mL	ricotta cheese (1 [16-oz./500 g] container)
4		eggs, lightly beaten
1 tsp.	5 mL	salt
¼ tsp.	1 mL	black pepper
12		full sheets phyllo pastry, defrosted

Preheat the oven to 350°F (180°C). Brush a 9 x 13–inch (23 x 33 cm) rectangular baking dish with melted butter.

Rinse the spinach and trim off any tough stems. Place it in a large pot or Dutch oven over medium-high heat. Cook, adding no additional water, just until the spinach is wilted, about 5 minutes.

Place the spinach in a colander and squeeze out as much of the liquid as possible. Chop coarsely and transfer to a bowl. Set aside.

Melt 1 tbsp. (15 mL) of the butter in a skillet over medium heat. Add the onion and cook, stirring, for about 5 minutes, until softened.

Add the chopped spinach and sauté for 1 to 2 minutes.

Phyllo Pastry: Easier Than You Think

Working with phyllo pastry isn't difficult as long as you remember to treat it with a little tender loving care. Take the package of frozen phyllo pastry out of the freezer the day before you want to use it and place it in the refrigerator to defrost. If you have forgotten to do this, don't try to defrost it at room temperature (or, worse, in the microwave). Just don't. Really.

When you are ready to use your phyllo, open the box and remove the sleeve containing the pastry. Unwrap it carefully, and then unfold the pastry leaves onto a dish towel. Work quickly, keeping the pastry covered with another dish towel to prevent it from drying out. (Because phyllo pastry is so thin, it dries out very quickly when exposed to air and becomes brittle and hard to handle.) If a sheet happens to tear as you're working with it, you can simply cover with another layer of phyllo to hide the split — no harm done.

When you are finished making your creation, re-roll any leftover pastry, slide it back into the plastic sleeve, seal it tightly and put it back into the freezer. Phyllo pastry can safely be refrozen.

Transfer the spinach mixture to a bowl and let cool for a few minutes. Add the feta, ricotta, eggs, salt and pepper. Mix well.

Melt the remaining butter in a small saucepan. Keep warm.

Now for the phyllo pastry. Remove the roll of pastry from the box and carefully unroll it (see box). Carefully remove 12 full sheets of phyllo and place them on a tray or dish towel on a flat surface. Cover with a second towel or sheet of plastic wrap. Immediately (quick, before you forget!) roll up the rest of the dough and return it to the package.

Now you're ready to assemble this masterpiece. Lay one sheet of phyllo on the bottom of the prepared baking dish, letting the extra climb up the sides. Brush with melted butter and lay another sheet of phyllo on top and brush again with butter.

Repeat this procedure until you have lined the bottom of the pan with 6 sheets of phyllo, each one brushed with butter.

Spread the spinach mixture over the phyllo in the dish.

Now cover the filling with a sheet of phyllo, letting the excess overhang the sides of the dish. Brush with butter, add another sheet, brush with butter (etc., etc., etc.) until you've used up the rest of the phyllo. There should be a total of six layers of phyllo on top of the spinach mixture.

Using a flexible rubber spatula, very gently tuck the excess overhanging pastry down along the sides of the baking dish, as if you were tucking sheets under a mattress. Brush the top with the remaining butter.

Place the spanakopita in the preheated oven and bake for 45 to 50 minutes, until the top is golden and the middle of the dish is slightly puffed. Serve hot or at room temperature.

Makes 6 to 8 servings.

An Appetizing Idea!

Use this same recipe to make little bite-sized spanakopita triangles. Here's how:

Cut each sheet of phyllo pastry into 4 lengthwise strips. Brush each strip with some melted butter, and then place 1 tbsp. (15 mL) of the filling at one end of the strip. Now fold it into triangles following the diagram below. Place on a greased baking sheet, brush the tops with butter and bake at 350°F (180°C) for 15 to 20 minutes, until golden brown and crisp.

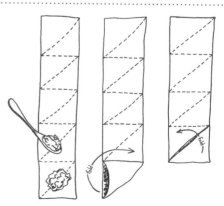

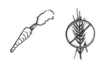

Oven-Roasted Carrot and Sweet Potato Casserole

A little sweet, a little exotic — this dish turns humble root vegetables and a can of chickpeas into a wonderful fall dinner.

4		medium onions, sliced
3 tbsp.	45 mL	olive oil or vegetable oil, divided
1 (19 oz.)	1 (540 mL)	can chickpeas, drained (or 2 cups/500 mL cooked dried chickpeas)
4		medium carrots, cut into ½-inch (1 cm) chunks
4		medium sweet potatoes, peeled and cut into ½-inch (1 cm) chunks
½ cup	125 mL	vegetable stock, homemade or store-bought (canned or from bouillon cubes or powder) or water
¼ cup	60 mL	raisins
¼ cup	60 mL	granulated sugar
½ tsp.	2 mL	cinnamon
½ tsp.	2 mL	salt
¼ tsp.	1 mL	black pepper

Preheat the oven to 400°F (200°C). Grease a 9 x 13–inch (23 x 33 cm) rectangular baking dish.

In a large skillet, sauté the onions in 2 tbsp. (30 mL) of the oil for 6 to 8 minutes, until softened and beginning to turn golden.

Spread evenly in the prepared baking dish. Sprinkle the chickpeas over the onions.

In a large bowl, toss together the carrots, sweet potatoes, stock or water, raisins, sugar, cinnamon, salt, pepper and the remaining 1 tbsp. (15 mL) of oil. Dump this over the chickpeas and spread it out evenly.

Place in the preheated oven and bake for 35 to 45 minutes, basting the top occasionally with some of the juices from the bottom of the baking dish, until the vegetables are tender and browned.

Makes 6 to 8 servings.

Spicy Quinoa with Black Beans and Corn

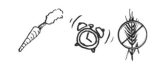

It's pronounced "keen-wa" and it's fantastic. Not only is it high in protein and quick to cook, quinoa also happens to be really delicious and versatile. You can use it instead of rice in many recipes or you can whip up this tasty quinoa main dish in a hurry.

1 tbsp.	15 mL	olive oil or vegetable oil
1		medium onion, chopped
2		cloves garlic, minced or pressed
1 cup	250 mL	quinoa, rinsed well and drained
1 tsp.	5 mL	cumin
¼ tsp.	1 mL	cayenne pepper, or more, if you like
¼ tsp.	1 mL	black pepper
1½ cups	375 mL	vegetable stock, homemade or store-bought (canned or from bouillon cubes or powder)
1 cup	250 mL	corn kernels, fresh or frozen
1 (19 oz.)	1 (540 mL)	can black beans, drained and rinsed
¼ cup	60 mL	fresh cilantro or parsley, chopped

Heat the oil in a medium saucepan over medium heat. Add the onion and garlic and cook, stirring, for about 5 minutes, until softened.

Add the quinoa, cumin, cayenne and pepper and stir for a few moments, to mix. Add the stock, stir and bring the mixture to a boil. Reduce the heat to low, cover the pot and simmer for 20 minutes. The quinoa should be tender and most of the liquid absorbed.

Add the corn and beans, stir to mix and then replace the cover and let cook for an additional 5 minutes, until everything is heated through.

Remove from the heat and let sit, covered, for 5 minutes, then sprinkle with the cilantro or parsley and serve immediately.

Makes 4 servings.

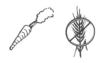

Paella with Tomatoes and Peas

This is a wonderful dish to make in late summer when tomatoes are in season and full of flavor. If you can get your hands on some Spanish smoked paprika, use it in this dish instead of regular paprika for extra awesomeness.

1½ lbs.	750 g	ripe tomatoes, cut into thick wedges (5 or 6 medium)
4 tbsp.	60 mL	olive oil, divided
½ tsp.	2 mL	salt, divided
¼ tsp.	1 mL	black pepper, divided
1		medium onion, chopped
4		cloves garlic, minced or pressed
1 tbsp.	15 mL	tomato paste
1 tbsp.	15 mL	paprika
2 cups	500 mL	Arborio rice
3½ cups	800 mL	vegetable stock, homemade or store-bought (canned or from bouillon cubes or powder), heated to steaming
1 cup	250 mL	fresh or frozen peas
		fresh parsley, chopped, for garnish.

Preheat oven to 450°F (230°C). Put the tomatoes in a medium bowl, sprinkle with 1 tbsp. (15 mL) of the olive oil and just a sprinkle of the salt and pepper (you'll use the rest later). Mix well and set aside.

Heat the remaining oil in a very large (12-inch/30 cm) ovenproof skillet over medium-high heat. Add the onion, garlic, salt and pepper and cook, stirring often, for about 5 minutes, until the onion is softened.

Stir in the tomato paste and paprika and cook for 1 to 2 minutes, just until blended.

Add the rice and cook for 1 to 2 minutes, stirring constantly, until the rice is shiny and everything is well mixed.

Add the stock and peas and stir to combine. Remove from the heat.

Arrange the tomato wedges on top of the rice in an artistic manner (or just carelessly, any which way — it doesn't matter, really).

Pour the tomato juices from the bowl over everything and put the pan into the preheated oven. Bake for 15 to 20 minutes, checking after 15 minutes to see if the rice is tender and most of the liquid has been absorbed. When it's done, turn off the oven but leave the pan inside for an additional 10 minutes to allow all the liquid to be absorbed. Sprinkle with chopped parsley and serve.

Makes 4 to 6 servings.

Split Cooking: A Survival Strategy for the Mixed Household

Perhaps someone you know and love (or like, anyway) has just turned vegetarian. Your first reaction might be annoyance. How dare they? You fear the worst, of course. Lentils. Brussels sprouts. Rutabaga. Tofu. There will be weird, inconvenient meals of strange foods from foreign countries. You are afraid that making dinner will take five hours. Calm down. It's not as scary as it seems. What you need is a strategy.

- When you dissect a typical meal, you'll usually find quite a few things that a vegetarian can eat. The vegetables, of course, and the rice, the salad, the bread. If the main dish is to be, for instance, a steak, this would clearly be your problem area. Easy enough. Just substitute something else: a veggie burger, perhaps (homemade or store-bought) or a vegetable pot pie. Make a bean stew, some chili or a meatless lasagna. Just divide it into portions and keep it in the freezer. You'll always have something ready to plunk on a plate instead of the meat.

- If you're making a stir-fry, cook the chicken or beef separately from the vegetables, and toss them together just at the end, having reserved a portion to be meatless. You can stir-fry some tofu or beans to add to the vegetarian version of the dish.

- Brown the hamburger for chili or spaghetti sauce separately and add it to the dish after a vegetarian portion has been removed. (Yes, the meat can be added later, just simmer it in the sauce for a little while before serving.) Substitute another protein, like crumbled tofu, tempeh, TVP or extra beans, to the veggie version. In fact, it wouldn't hurt for everyone to double up on the vegetables.

- Keep the fridge stocked with firm tofu, which easily lends itself to meat-like cooking techniques. Marinate it in barbecue sauce and bake it, grill it, bread it and panfry it, or simmer it in the same sauce you're using to cook the chicken.

- Designate a couple of days of the week as non-meat for everyone. Experiment with vegetarian versions of familiar dishes — pizza, lasagna, tacos. You may even like them better that way.

- Encourage your resident vegetarian to cook. Have him or her plan the meals and prepare some or all of the dishes. You'll broaden your horizons while splitting the workload. Not a bad plan, on the whole.

Deeply Personal Pizzas

Each of the pizzas in this section begins with a homemade crust using half of a recipe for Ultra-Quick All-Purpose Yeast Dough (see page 188). But since you know you'll want to have pizza again soon, go ahead and make the full batch of dough. You can either make two pizzas (and freeze one for later or eat both now) or you can just pop the extra ball of dough into the freezer so it's ready to use another time. Prepared frozen dough just needs to be defrosted and rolled out before using.

Pizza with Tomato Sauce and Whatever

Here's an old pizza-maker's trick for making a vegetable pizza with cheese: sauce first, then cheese, then the veggies on top of the cheese. This allows the steam from the vegetables to escape and prevents sogginess. Try it for yourself.

½		recipe Ultra-Quick All-Purpose Yeast Dough (see page 188) or 1 (12-inch/30 cm) unbaked pizza crust
1 cup	250 mL	All-Purpose Tomato Sauce (see page 95) or store-bought tomato pasta sauce
2 cups	500 mL	shredded mozzarella cheese
		additional toppings (see below if you need inspiration)

Preheat the oven to 450°F (230°C). Grease a 12-inch (30 cm) pizza pan (a cookie sheet will do). Sprinkle the pan with cornmeal.

On a well-floured surface, roll out the dough to a 12-inch (30 cm) round. Transfer to the prepared pan and pinch the edges up to form a bit of a ridge around the edge.

Spread the pasta sauce evenly over the crust in the baking pan, to about ½ inch (1 cm) from the edge.

Sprinkle with the shredded mozzarella cheese, then top with whatever toppings you want to use.

Place in the preheated oven and bake for about 20 to 25 minutes, until the cheese is bubbling and the crust is browned when you peek underneath.

Makes one 12-inch (30 cm) pizza or 3 to 4 servings. Or less.

Pizza Topping Ideas (Some Obvious, Some Not So Obvious)

- Sliced fresh mushrooms
- Chopped green or red sweet peppers
- Chopped or sliced onions
- Diced or sliced fresh tomatoes
- Sliced grilled eggplant
- Chopped sun-dried tomatoes
- Torn fresh basil leaves
- Broccoli florets
- Chopped roasted red peppers
- Chopped fresh hot peppers or prepared hot pepper rings
- Chopped or sliced marinated artichoke hearts
- Sliced green or black olives
- Fresh or frozen corn kernels
- Thinly sliced potatoes
- Pineapple chunks (to each his own)

Do-It-Yourself Frozen Pizza

If you decide to make two pizzas at once and freeze the extra one for a rainy day, here's how to do it. Place the prepared, unbaked pizza in a pan and place in the freezer — don't cover it or anything. Let freeze solid, then lift it from the pan and wrap it tightly in foil or plastic; because it's frozen it won't stick to the wrappings. To bake, remove from the freezer and unwrap. Place on a lightly greased pan and bake at 450°F (230°C) for 25 to 30 minutes, or until done the way you like it. You are so clever.

Pizza with Pesto, Goat Cheese and Sun-Dried Tomatoes

Make your own pesto sauce (see page 96) or use store-bought for this deliciously different pizza. You may never go back to tomato sauce again.

½		recipe Ultra-Quick All-Purpose Yeast Dough (see page 188) or 1 (12-inch/30 cm) unbaked pizza crust
1 cup	250 mL	pesto sauce, homemade (see page 96) or store-bought
½ cup	125 mL	oil-packed sun-dried tomatoes, drained and cut into strips
5 oz.	140 g	goat cheese, plain or with herbs, crumbled (about 1 cup/250 mL)

Preheat the oven to 450°F (230°C). Grease a 12-inch (30 cm) pizza pan, or if you don't have an official one, a cookie sheet will do. Sprinkle the pan with cornmeal.

On a well-floured surface, roll out the dough to a 12-inch (30 cm) round. Transfer to the prepared pan and pinch the edges up to form a bit of a ridge around the edge.

Spread the pesto sauce evenly over the prepared pizza crust to about ½-inch (1 cm) from the edge.

Sprinkle with the sun-dried tomatoes and top with crumbled goat cheese.

Bake in the preheated oven for about 25 minutes, until the pesto is sizzling and the crust is browned when you peek underneath.

Makes one 12-inch (30 cm) pizza or 3 to 4 servings. Or less.

Pizza with Caramelized Onions and Pine Nuts

Sweet caramelized onions, creamy goat cheese, crunchy pine nuts. This is one amazing pizza. Prepare to become famous.

1 tbsp.	15 mL	olive oil
1 tbsp.	15 mL	butter
3		medium onions, thinly sliced
2 tbsp.	30 mL	balsamic vinegar
1 tbsp.	15 mL	granulated sugar
½ tsp.	2 mL	salt
½		recipe Ultra-Quick All-Purpose Yeast Dough (see page 188) or 1 (12-inch/30 cm) unbaked pizza crust
5 oz.	140 g	goat cheese, plain or with herbs, crumbled (about 1 cup/250 mL)
¼ cup	60 mL	pine nuts

First, make the caramelized onions. Heat the olive oil and butter (you can use all olive oil, if you prefer) in a large skillet over medium-low heat. Add the sliced onions and cook, stirring occasionally, until the onions turn a deep golden brown, about 30 minutes.

Add the balsamic vinegar, sugar and salt and cook for 5 minutes, until the liquid has almost completely evaporated. Let cool.

Preheat the oven to 450°F (230°C). Grease a 12-inch (30 cm) pizza pan, or if you don't have an official one, a cookie sheet will do. Sprinkle the pan with cornmeal.

On a well-floured surface, roll out the dough to a 12-inch (30 cm) round. Transfer to the prepared pan and pinch the edges up to form a bit of a ridge around the edge.

Smoosh the goat cheese, as evenly as possible, over the prepared pizza crust to about ½ inch (1 cm) from the edge.

Spread the onions over the cheese, then sprinkle with the pine nuts.

Bake in the preheated oven for about 25 minutes, until the top is sizzling and the crust is browned when you peek underneath.

Makes 2 to 3 servings. Or maybe just one…

Five More Brilliant Pizza Possibilities

- Very thinly sliced potatoes, thinly sliced red onion, crumbled blue cheese and fresh rosemary.
- Fresh spinach leaves, roasted red peppers, chopped onion and feta cheese.
- Grilled or broiled eggplant slices, diced fresh tomato, chopped garlic and ricotta cheese.
- Sautéed sliced portobello mushrooms with garlic, mozzarella cheese and Parmesan.
- Spicy Mexican salsa, corn kernels and Monterey Jack cheese.

Roasted Red Peppers

When red peppers are in season you can often buy beautiful ones quite cheaply. This is the time to make a big batch of roasted red peppers to freeze. You may not feel like doing it right now, but in February, when a red pepper can cost as much as a month's rent, you'll be so happy to have these stashed away.

Cut the peppers in half lengthwise through the stem end, and remove the seeds and the spongy stuff inside. If you have a barbecue, place the peppers skin-side down on the grill and roast them until the skin turns black. Totally.

If you don't have access to a barbecue, just arrange the seeded pepper halves skin-side up on a baking sheet in the oven and broil close to the element until black.

When your peppers are well charred, toss them into a covered container or a plastic bag and let them steam for a few minutes until they're cool enough to handle. Now peel away the blackened skin, it should be easy to remove, and place the peppers on a plastic-lined cookie sheet. Put the cookie sheet in the freezer and let the peppers freeze solid, and then peel them off the plastic, pack them into plastic bags and put them back into the freezer.

Congratulations, you are now the proud owner of a whole bunch of individually frozen roasted red peppers. They can be chopped and tossed with cooked pasta or rice, slivered into a salad or layered on a sandwich.

Random Delights

Baked Barbecue Tofu Steaks

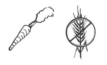

This is a tofu recipe for people who think they don't like tofu. The extra-firm tofu holds up beautifully when baked with a flavorful sauce and has a texture that appeals to the newly vegetarianized. Exact package size may vary slightly, depending on the brand — anything close will do.

1 (12 oz.)	1 (350 g)	package extra-firm tofu
1 cup	250 mL	barbecue sauce, any kind you like (try honey garlic or teriyaki)

Cut tofu into ½-inch (1 cm) thick slices and place in bowl or baking dish.

Add the barbecue sauce and turn the slices over to coat them on all sides.

Cover the bowl or dish and place in the refrigerator and allow the tofu to marinate for at least 1 hour or, for maximum flavor, overnight.

Preheat the oven to 375°F (190°C). Grease a 9 x 13–inch (23 x 33 cm) rectangular baking dish.

Dump the marinated tofu and all the sauce into the prepared baking dish and arrange the slices in a single layer.

Bake in the preheated oven for about 30 minutes, turning the slices over a few times and basting with the sauce, until the tofu is sizzling and well glazed. Remove from oven and serve with rice, potatoes, bread or something that will soak up the sauce.

Makes 2 or 3 servings.

Breaded Tofu Fingers

Vegetarian fish sticks, really. Great kid food — or adult food, for that matter. Don't forget the dipping sauce.

1 (12 oz.)	1 (350 g)	package extra-firm tofu
½ cup	125 mL	dry bread crumbs
¼ tsp.	1 mL	salt
¼ tsp.	1 mL	black pepper
¼ tsp.	1 mL	crumbled dried oregano
¼ tsp.	1 mL	garlic powder
¼ cup	60 mL	all-purpose white or whole-wheat flour
1		egg, beaten
		your favorite dipping sauces

Preheat the oven to 375°F (190°C). Grease a cookie sheet.

Cut the block of tofu into fingers about ½ inch (1 cm) thick and 3 inches (8 cm) long, more or less.

In a small bowl, combine the bread crumbs, salt, pepper, oregano and garlic powder. Place the flour in another small bowl. Have the beaten egg ready in a third bowl.

First toss the tofu fingers in the flour, then dip each one into the beaten egg and then roll in the bread crumb mixture. (The flour step, by the way, helps bind the egg and crumbs to the tofu, so that the crumbs don't just fall off.)

Place breaded fingers on the prepared cookie sheet and bake in the preheated oven for about 30 minutes, turning them over halfway through.

Veggie Dogs and Other Pretend Meats

Vegetarian meat substitutes are usually sold in packages in a refrigerated supermarket case near the cheeses or in the produce section. These are generally made from soy protein, processed to resemble various meat products, such as hot dogs, hamburger patties, ground beef or chicken. They can often be used as a straight substitute for the real thing in many meat-based recipes and can be especially useful for vegetarians just learning to cook meatless.

These pretend meat products may have twice as much (or sometimes more) protein, percentagewise, as in a comparable amount of actual meat, are generally lower in fat and, of course, contain no cholesterol.

For a new vegetarian (is that you?) or for vegetarian kids who want to appear to be eating what all their friends are eating, these products are ideal. They're also great when you are faced with feeding carnivorous friends or family members who are afraid that they will have to eat weird food at your house.

Serve the tofu fingers hot with an assortment of dipping sauces: ketchup, sweet and sour, plum sauce, barbecue sauce, hot mustard, whatever.

Makes about 16 fingers.

Tofu Veggie Kebabs with Peanut Sauce

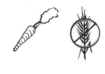

Make these tasty skewers for your next barbecue and you'll have all the carnivores begging for a taste. Go ahead, share. It's the right thing to do.

1 recipe		Peanut Sauce from Spicy Peanut Pasta (see page 104)
1 (12 oz.)	1 (350 g)	package extra-firm tofu
1		medium red or green sweet pepper, cut into 1-inch (2 cm) squares
1		medium onion, cut into 1-inch (2 cm) chunks
1		medium zucchini, cut into 1-inch (2 cm) chunks
½ lb.	250 g	mushrooms, cut in half or leave whole, if small (about 2½ cups/625 mL)

Place the tofu cubes in a bowl and add about half the peanut sauce. Stir to mix, cover the bowl with plastic wrap and refrigerate for at least 30 minutes or as long as overnight. Cover and refrigerate the remaining peanut sauce.

Soak 10 bamboo skewers in water for at least 30 minutes.

When you're ready to cook, fish the marinated tofu cubes out of the sauce and spear them on the soaked skewers alternately with the vegetables (in any order you like) until all the tofu and vegetables are used up. Hang onto the marinade.

Preheat the barbecue grill to medium heat. Place the kebabs on the grill and cook, brushing several times with the reserved marinade and turning to cook all sides evenly. The tofu should be browned and sizzling and the vegetables tender but still crisp.

Serve the kebabs over rice or noodles, drizzled with the remaining peanut sauce.

Makes 4 servings.

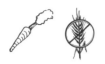

Baked Stuffed Portobello Mushrooms

Portobello mushrooms are, basically, the steak of the vegetable world. Serve one of these per person as a side dish or light main dish or two per person for a hearty dinner.

Other Stuffing Suggestions

- Add a handful of chopped fresh spinach or shredded zucchini to pan with the onions and carrots.
- Add 1 cup (250 mL) shredded mozzarella or cheddar cheese along with the rice.
- Try stuffing these mushrooms with the same mixture your Aunt Dorothy uses in her Thanksgiving turkey. (You'll have to phone her to get the recipe.)
- Instead of the brown rice in this recipe, try cooked orzo, quinoa, couscous or any small pasta.

4		medium-sized portobello mushrooms
1 tbsp.	15 mL	olive oil or vegetable oil, plus more for drizzling
1		medium onion, finely chopped
1		clove garlic, minced or pressed
1		medium carrot, finely chopped
½		green sweet pepper, finely chopped
1 cup	250 mL	cooked brown rice (see page 163)
1 tbsp.	15 mL	fresh basil, chopped (or 1 tsp./5 mL dried)
1 tsp.	5 mL	crumbled dried oregano
1 tsp.	5 mL	salt
¼ tsp.	1 mL	black pepper
		grated Parmesan cheese for sprinkling, if desired

Preheat the oven to 400°F (200°C). Grease a 9-inch (23 cm) square baking dish.

Rinse the mushroom caps or wipe with a paper towel to remove any dirt. Cut the stems from the caps and chop the stems finely. Set the caps aside.

Heat the oil in a large skillet over medium heat. Add the chopped mushroom stems, the onion, garlic, carrot and green pepper. Cook, stirring, for 6 to 8 minutes, until the vegetables are softened.

Remove from heat and stir in the rice, basil, oregano, salt and pepper.

Arrange the mushrooms gill-side up in the prepared baking dish. Fill caps with the rice mixture, dividing it equally among the mushrooms and packing it down lightly. Drizzle the tops with a bit more oil and sprinkle with Parmesan cheese (if desired).

Place in the preheated oven and bake for 20 to 30 minutes, until the mushrooms are tender and the stuffing is hot. Serve immediately.

Makes 2 main dish or 4 side dish servings.

Grilled Marinated Portobello Mushrooms

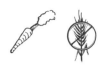

Thick, juicy, meaty. These mushrooms were born to be grilled. Serve them as "burgers" in a bun with all the trimmings or on a plate as a delicious mushroom steak.

4		large portobello mushroom caps
½ cup	125 mL	olive oil
¼ cup	60 mL	balsamic vinegar
2 tbsp.	30 mL	fresh parsley, chopped
2		cloves garlic, squished
½ tsp.	2 mL	salt
¼ tsp.	1 mL	pepper

Rinse mushroom caps or wipe with a paper towel to remove any dirt. Remove the stems (save these for your stock bag, see page 39). Place the caps in a clean zipper-top plastic bag.

In a small bowl, whisk together the olive oil, balsamic vinegar, parsley, garlic, salt and pepper. Pour into the bag with the mushroom caps.

Press out as much of the air from the bag as possible and zip the top shut. Refrigerate and let the mushrooms marinate for 4 to 6 hours.

When you're ready to cook, preheat the barbecue grill to medium-high heat.

Remove the mushroom caps from the bag and place on the preheated barbecue grill, cap-side up. Grill until the caps begin to soften, about 5 minutes, basting occasionally with marinade. Flip the mushrooms over and grill cap-side down until hot and sizzling and the mushroom juice has pooled in the caps.

Remove carefully from the barbecue, taking care not to lose any of the delicious juice, and place each cap on a warm, toasted hamburger bun. Top with whatever you like (sliced onions, tomatoes, hot peppers, shredded mozzarella, lettuce, you know) and eat.

Share nicely, now. Isn't that why you made extra?

Makes 4 servings.

Fabulous Side Dish Idea!

Grill portobello mushrooms as above but instead of serving them on a bun, slice them crosswise about ¼ inch (0.5 cm) thick and serve as an appetizer or side dish with crusty bread to sop up the delicious mushroom juices. Who wouldn't love this?

Tofu Veggie Burgers

Make a batch of these burgers and freeze them on a baking sheet lined with waxed paper. They're better and cheaper than store-bought veggie burgers, and since you made them yourself, you know exactly what's in them.

1 (12 oz.)	1 (350 g)	package extra-firm tofu, frozen and thawed
¼ cup	60 mL	olive oil or vegetable oil
1		medium onion, chopped
½ lb.	250 g	mushrooms, chopped (about 2½ cups/625 mL)
1		medium carrot, grated
1½ cups	375 mL	cooked brown rice
1½ cups	375 mL	bread crumbs
½ cup	125 mL	barbecue sauce (any kind; a smoky flavor is nice)
2 tbsp.	30 mL	cornstarch
1 tsp.	5 mL	salt
¼ tsp.	1 mL	black pepper
1 cup	250 mL	frozen peas or corn (or some of each), thawed
2		eggs

By hand, squeeze as much of the water out of the thawed tofu as possible and crumble it finely into a large bowl.

Heat the oil in a medium skillet, add the chopped onion and mushrooms and cook until all of the liquid has evaporated and the mixture is beginning to brown slightly. This will take about 8 to 10 minutes.

Add to the crumbled tofu in the bowl. Add the grated carrot, rice, bread crumbs, barbecue sauce, cornstarch, salt and pepper. Mix gently.

Put the thawed peas or corn (or both) into the container of a blender or food processor along with the eggs. Whirl until the eggs are beaten and the corn and peas are chopped. Add to the mixture in the bowl, and stir until everything is very well combined.

Wet your hands and form the burger mixture into patties, using about ½ cup (125 mL) for each patty. Flatten into a burger shape and place on a wax paper–lined tray. You should end up with about eight burgers.

To grill your burgers, preheat the barbecue on high heat. Place a grill-top rack (it looks like a griddle, but with holes that keeps small things from falling into the burners) on the barbecue grid.

Brush burgers on both sides with oil and grill until well browned on both sides, flipping over once. If you want, you can brush the cooked side with a bit of barbecue sauce as it continues to cook. Serve in a fresh hamburger bun with lots of the usual stuff.

To bake your burgers, place on an oiled cookie sheet and bake at 375°F (190°C) for about 30 minutes, turning them over halfway through. Serve as above.

Or, finally, you can simply pan fry them in a bit of vegetable oil, turning over to cook both sides. And ditto on the serving suggestions.

Makes about 8 burgers.

Mostly Mushroom Burgers

This recipe works well with any kind of fresh mushroom, but especially the bargain-bin ones that are just a little past their prime. Pick up a bunch and make these. Mushrooms should be fairly finely chopped (but not pureed) — a food processor works wonders here.

2 tbsp.	30 ml	olive oil or vegetable oil
1½ lbs.	750 g	fresh mushrooms, chopped (white, cremini, portobellos or a mixture)
½		medium onion, minced
2		cloves garlic, minced or pressed
¾ cup	175 mL	bread crumbs
⅔ cup	150 mL	rolled oats
½ cup	125 mL	grated Parmesan cheese
2		eggs, beaten
1 tsp.	5 ml	salt
¼ tsp.	1 mL	black pepper

Heat the oil in a large skillet over medium-high heat. Add the chopped mushrooms, onion and garlic and cook, stirring often, for about 10 minutes, until the mushrooms have released all their liquid and it has evaporated. Transfer to a medium bowl. Let cool for a few minutes.

Add the bread crumbs, oats, Parmesan cheese, eggs, salt and pepper. Mix until all the ingredients are evenly combined and mushy. Cover and refrigerate for at least 15 minutes or as long as overnight. The mixture becomes stickier as it sits, good if you want your burgers to hold together.

Marvellous Mushroom Meatballs!

This same recipe can be used to make delicious mushroom meatballs. Roll mushroom mixture into 1-inch (2 cm) balls and place on a well-oiled cookie sheet. Brush the tops with more oil. Bake at 375°F (190°C) for 15 minutes, turn them over and continue to bake for another 10 to 15 minutes, until sizzling and browned. Simmer for just a few minutes in basic pasta sauce or any other place a regular meatball might be found.

Form the mushroom mixture into four patties no more than ½ inch (1 cm) thick.

Now you have options… To grill, preheat the barbecue on high heat. Place a grill-top rack (it looks like a griddle, but with holes that keeps small things from falling into the burners) on the barbecue grid. Brush mushroom burgers on both sides with oil and grill until well browned on both sides, flipping over once.

To panfry, pour 1 tbsp. (15 mL) of oil into a skillet and place over medium-high heat until hot. Cook burgers on both sides until well browned.

Serve mushroom burgers on a bun with all the usual burger accompaniments — and let the carnivores beg for a taste. Be nice — let them have some.

Makes 4 burgers.

Yikes! I Didn't Know There Was Meat in There!

Beneath the seemingly vegetarian facade of many prepared food products lurks meat, fish and other non-vegetarian ingredients. It can be in the form of animal fat (like lard or beef fat), meat extracts or stock (chicken or beef stock–based vegetable soups) or even seafood (fish extracts in pad thai). The only way to be sure you're not eating this stuff is to become an obsessive label-reader. Here are a few surprises you might never have considered:

- Packaged crackers (even plain ones) may be made with animal fat (lard or beef fat).

- Some brands of cookies are made with animal fats like lard or beef fat.

- Vegetable lasagna may contain meat-based stock.

- Canned chili-style beans may be made with lard.

- Fruit-flavored jelly powder is made with gelatin, an animal extract.

- Many brands of yogurt contain gelatin (see above).

- Some bottled stir-fry sauces contain oyster sauce, which is, yes, made from oysters.

- Even a non-meat commercial spaghetti sauce may contain beef or chicken extract or stock.

- Canned vegetable soup may contain chicken or beef stock unless specifically labeled otherwise.

- Worcestershire sauce contains anchovies (okay, so that's a fish, but still).

Messy Josephines

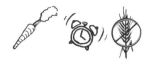

A slightly more refined, vegetarian version of the classic meat-based Sloppy Joe.

1 cup	250 mL	TVP granules
2 tbsp.	30 mL	soy sauce
¾ cup	175 mL	hot water
3 tbsp.	45 mL	olive oil or vegetable oil
½ lb.	250 g	mushrooms, chopped (2½ cups/625 mL)
1		medium onion, chopped
1		stalk celery, chopped
¼ cup	60 mL	vegetable stock, homemade or store-bought (canned or from bouillon cubes or powder)
¼ cup	60 mL	ketchup or barbecue sauce
½ tsp.	2 mL	hot pepper sauce (or more, or less, or none)

Put the TVP in a medium bowl.

In a measuring cup, stir together the hot water and soy sauce.

Pour over the TVP in the bowl, stir and set the TVP aside to soak and rehydrate while you prepare the rest of the ingredients.

Heat the oil in a large skillet over medium heat. Add the mushrooms, onion and celery and cook, stirring, for 6 to 8 minutes, until the mushrooms are tender and they have released their juices.

Add the rehydrated TVP to the vegetable mixture in the skillet. Let cook for 5 to 7 minutes, and then stir in the vegetable stock, ketchup and hot pepper sauce. Simmer the mixture, stirring, for about 5 minutes, until the flavors are blended and everything is nicely gloppy.

Spoon over 4 split, toasted hamburger buns and eat. Messily.

Makes 4 sandwiches

Messy Josephine Goes Tofu!

Instead of the TVP in this recipe, you can use a block of extra-firm tofu that was frozen, then thawed, squeezed out by hand and crumbled. Add to the vegetables in the pan, along with 2 tbsp. (30 mL) soy sauce.

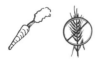

Tempeh Teriyaki

This is similar enough meat to make a vegetarian feel, well, uncomfortable. Relax, it's just soybeans. See below for details.

1 (8.5 oz.)	1 (240 g)	package tempeh
⅓ cup	75 mL	soy sauce
2 tbsp.	30 mL	brown sugar
2 tbsp.	30 mL	rice vinegar, cider vinegar or lemon juice
1 tbsp.	15 mL	vegetable oil
2		cloves garlic, minced or pressed
1 tsp.	5 mL	fresh ginger root, finely grated

Cut the block of tempeh into ½-inch (1 cm) cubes. Place in a steamer basket over boiling water, and steam for 20 minutes. Remove to a bowl.

In a small bowl, mix together the soy sauce, brown sugar, vinegar or lemon juice, oil, garlic and ginger. Pour this mixture over the tempeh and stir to coat the cubes evenly. Cover, refrigerate and let marinate for at least 2 hours or overnight.

When you're ready to cook, preheat the broiler element in the oven. Grease a cookie sheet or broiler-safe baking dish.

Arrange the tempeh cubes on the prepared baking dish. Spoon the marinade over the cubes and place under the preheated broiler.

Broil until the tempeh is sizzling and glazed with the marinade, turning the cubes over to cook all sides. Watch carefully! The sugar in the sauce can cause it to burn easily.

Remove from the oven and serve tempeh and sauce spooned over rice or noodles as a main dish, or serve the cubes on toothpicks as an appetizer.

Makes 4 servings as a main dish.

Tempeh

Look, tempeh is unusual stuff, there's no doubt about it. A traditional Indonesian food, tempeh is made from soybeans that have been partially cooked, mixed with a bacterial culture (think yogurt) and then pressed into slabs and allowed to ferment. After a while, the tempeh is frozen to stop the fermentation. Tempeh is, therefore, most commonly sold as a frozen product.

As a result of this rather complicated process, tempeh develops an interesting, mushroomy flavor, a chewy texture and becomes highly digestible. After an initial steaming, tempeh can be diced and thrown into a stir-fry, baked or grilled with barbecue sauce or just chopped up, mixed with stuff and eaten as a salad or sandwich filling. It is an excellent source of protein, high in fiber and contains both calcium and B vitamins.

Full-Meal Burritos

This is no small snack. This is a fully loaded, knife-and-fork burrito that will make you very happy.

2 tbsp.	30 mL	olive oil or vegetable oil
4		cloves garlic, squished
3		green onions, finely chopped
1		red or green sweet pepper, chopped
1 or 2		jalapeño peppers, minced
1 (10 oz.)	1 (284 g)	package fresh spinach leaves (or about 6 cups/1.5 L loose leaves)
2 (19 oz)	2 (540 mL)	cans black beans, drained (or 4 cups/1 L cooked dried beans)
½ tsp.	2 mL	salt
¼ tsp.	1 mL	black pepper
4		large (10-inch/25 cm) flour tortillas, warmed
2 cups	500 mL	warm cooked white or brown rice or Mexican red rice (see page X)
2		medium tomatoes, diced
2 cups	500 mL	shredded Monterey Jack or cheddar cheese
		salsa, for serving
		sour cream, for serving

Heat the oil in a large skillet over medium heat. Add the garlic, green onions, sweet pepper and jalapeño and cook, stirring, for 6 to 8 minutes, until the vegetables are softened.

Add the spinach and continue to cook until the spinach is wilted, then add the black beans, salt and pepper. Cook, stirring occasionally, for about 5 minutes, until everything is combined.

To assemble, place a warm tortilla on a plate, add a spoonful of rice and a big scoop of the bean mixture. Top it with a sprinkle of shredded cheese and some chopped tomatoes, if using. Fold over the bottom and top then roll in the sides and place, seam-side down, on a plate. Serve immediately with salsa and sour cream on the side.

Sorry, but you'll probably need a knife and fork for these.

Makes 4 large burritos.

Sandwiches Galore

We all know how to make a sandwich, right? You get two slices of bread, smear with some butter, mayo or mustard and slap on whatever you've got in the house. Sometimes this will be excellent — nice cheese, crisp lettuce, fresh tomatoes, some lovely leftovers. Other times, however, there will be nothing. Well, nothing at first glance anyway. But if you use your imagination, you may just invent something wonderful. Here are just a few suggestions to get you started.

On a Fresh Bun:

- Egg salad — regular or tofu (see page 66).
- Sautéed or grilled mushrooms with cheese and tomato.
- Grilled eggplant and peppers drizzled with olive oil and balsamic vinegar.

Stuffed into a Pita Pocket:

- Hummus and mixed green salad.
- Eggplant Caviar (see page 26) and crumbled feta cheese.
- Diced avocado, shredded cheese and tomato (with a dab of mayonnaise).
- Chickpea Curry (see page 123).
- Diced tomato, mozzarella cheese and arugula drizzled with a bit of olive oil.
- Scrambled Tofu (see page 88) with diced tomatoes and lettuce.

Open-Faced:

- Arrange slices of Swiss cheese and ripe pear on toast and broil until the cheese melts.
- Spread tomato sauce on a toasted English muffin, sprinkle with cheese and broil.
- Cream cheese, honey, walnuts and chopped apple on slices of whole-wheat toast.
- Bruschetta mixture (see page 24) on garlic toast.

Folded into a Tortilla:

- Cuban-Style Black Beans (see page 131), shredded cheese and lettuce.
- Potato and Green Pea Curry (see page 124).
- Peanut butter, banana and honey.
- Leftover chili.

Cream Cheese Combos:

- Peanut butter, cream cheese and honey (with or without banana) on whole-wheat bread.
- Cream cheese, sliced hard-boiled eggs, pickles and alfalfa sprouts in a pita pocket.
- Cream cheese mixed with shredded cheddar, celery and chives on a toasted English muffin.
- Cream cheese, raisins and cashews on multigrain bread.

7. Sidekicks

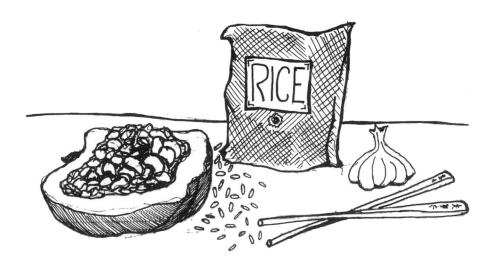

All Kinds of Grains: The Basics

We'll start with rice — it's eaten all over the world and is just about the most versatile grain there is. And then we'll go from there. So many different grains to know and love.

Rice

As a vegetarian, you're bound to run into rice a lot, so you may as well learn to cook it well. Lucky for you, this is easy to do.

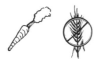

White Rice

All white rice is not the same. There are long-grain, short-grain and medium-grain varieties of white rice. There is Indian basmati rice, Thai jasmine rice and Italian Arborio rice. There is also converted rice. So how do you know what to use? Well, the long answer is that you'll have to experiment. Buy small quantities of different kinds of rice at a bulk food store and try each of them to see which ones you like best. They will differ from one another in flavor, texture and aroma, and each one is best used in a specific way. But never mind all that. If you keep a few different kinds on hand — Thai jasmine, Indian basmati and Italian Arborio — you'll always have the right rice to use when you need it. If no type has been specified in a recipe, you can usually get away with jasmine or basmati rice.

| 1 cup | 250 mL | white rice |
| 1½ cups | 375 mL | water |

Pour the water into a medium saucepan with a tight-fitting lid. Bring it to a boil over high heat. Add the rice to the boiling water and give it a stir. Reduce the heat to the barest simmer and cover the pot with the lid. Let cook for 15 minutes without peeking.

After 15 minutes, lift the lid and have a look. The water should be completely absorbed and the surface of the rice should look as if there are holes all over it. Don't stir, but taste a grain or two to see if the rice is tender. If it's not quite cooked, replace the lid and give it another 5 minutes then taste a grain again.

When the rice is cooked, remove the pan from the heat and let stand, covered, for about 5 minutes, then fluff with a fork and serve.

Makes about 3 cups (750 mL).

Brown Rice

Brown rice is rice that's still wearing an overcoat. The outer bran layer has been left on the grain, giving it a chewy texture, a nutty flavor and more vitamins and fiber than white rice. It takes a little longer to cook but, nutritionally speaking, it's a superior food. Brown rice goes especially well with hearty stews and beans. There are many varieties of brown rice, but the most common are short or medium-grain brown rice and brown basmati rice. Use whichever one you like best.

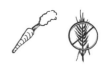

1 cup	250 mL	brown rice
2½ cups	625 mL	water

Pour the water into a medium saucepan with a tight-fitting lid. Bring it to a boil over high heat. Add the rice to the boiling water and give it a stir. Reduce the heat to the barest simmer and cover with the lid. Let cook for 35 minutes without peeking.

After 35 minutes, lift the lid and have a look. The water should be completely absorbed and the surface of the rice should look as if there are holes all over it. Don't stir, but taste a grain or two to see if the rice is tender. If it's not quite cooked, replace the lid and let it cook for another 5 to 10 minutes, then taste again.

When the rice is cooked, remove the pan from the heat and let stand, covered, for about 5 minutes, then fluff with a fork and serve.

Makes about 3 cups (750 mL).

Coconut Rice

The perfect partner to Cuban-Style Black Beans (see page 131) or any other spicy, saucy concoction. Nothing could be easier or more delicious.

Instead of water as the cooking liquid for your rice, substitute half water and half canned coconut milk. Add a pinch of salt. Otherwise follow the recipe as written and, voilà, perfect coconut rice. You can use regular or light (lower fat) coconut milk, either one will work.

Other Grains for Your Repertoire

Looking for something a little different to serve with that vegetable stew or chili? All of these basic grains are as easy to cook as rice and can be served alone, instead of pasta, rice or potatoes, or added to a pilaf or salad.

Barley

Serve plain with a stew, chilled in a salad or mixed with other grains as a side dish. Barley has a satisfyingly chewy texture that can stand up to practically anything. Pearl barley cooks more quickly than pot barley, but either one can be used.

| 1 cup | 250 mL | barley |
| 3 cups | 750 mL | water |

In a medium saucepan with a tight-fitting lid, combine the barley and water. Bring to a boil, uncovered, over high heat. Reduce the heat to low, cover the pan and cook until all the water has been absorbed and the barley is tender, about 35 to 45 minutes. When the barley is cooked, remove the pan from heat and let stand, covered, for 5 minutes. Fluff with a fork and serve immediately or rinse under cold running water to use cold in a salad.

Makes about 4 cups (1 L).

Quinoa

This tasty little grain is packed with protein and full of calcium and other minerals. A relative newcomer to this part of the world, quinoa was a staple of the ancient Incan diet. Unless the package says your quinoa has already been pre-rinsed, it will require a thorough rinsing before cooking to remove a natural coating that can cause the grain to taste soapy.

| 1 cup | 250 mL | quinoa |
| 1½ cups | 375 mL | water |

Rinse the dry quinoa well in several changes of water to remove the soapy coating on the grain. If not removed, this can give the cooked quinoa a bitter taste. (You can skip this step if the package says that the grain has been pre-rinsed.)

In a medium saucepan with a tight-fitting lid, combine the quinoa and water and bring to a boil over high heat. Reduce the heat to low, cover the pot and let simmer for 15 to 20 minutes, until all the liquid has been absorbed. Remove from the heat and let stand for about 5 minutes. Fluff with a fork and serve.

Makes 2½ cups (625 mL).

Bulgur Wheat

Bulgur is a form of whole wheat that has been partially cooked, then dehydrated and cracked into small granules. Because it's pre-cooked, bulgur only needs to be soaked in boiling water before using. Bulgur makes a mean tabbouleh salad (see page 74), but it can also be cooked as a pilaf (see page 170).

1 cup	250 mL	bulgur wheat
2 cups	500 mL	water

Put the bulgur in a bowl or saucepan. Bring the water to a boil and add to the bulgur in the bowl. Stir, then cover the bowl and let stand until the water has been absorbed, about 5 to 10 minutes. The bulgur will be chewy but tender and can be used in a salad, added to a soup or stew or seasoned to taste and served as a side dish.

Makes about 3 cups (750 mL).

Kasha

Kasha is just another name for buckwheat. It's sold in two forms, toasted or untoasted. This recipe calls for toasted kasha, which has a nutty, earthy flavor and goes well with mushrooms and saucy stews.

2 tbsp.	30 mL	olive oil or vegetable oil
2		medium onions, chopped
1		egg, beaten
1 cup	250 mL	toasted kasha
2 cups	500 mL	vegetable stock, homemade or store-bought (canned or from bouillon cubes or powder) or water
½ tsp.	2 mL	salt
¼ tsp.	1 mL	black pepper

Measure the oil into a medium saucepan with a tight-fitting lid. Place over medium heat, add the onions and cook, stirring often, for 8 to 10 minutes, until golden. Remove the onions from the pan and set aside.

In a small bowl, stir together the egg and the kasha. Dump into the same saucepan in which you sautéed the onions; no additional oil is needed. Cook, stirring to break up clumps, until the egg has coated the kasha and the grains are separate and beginning to brown slightly, about 5 minutes.

Add the stock or water and bring the mixture to a boil.

Stir in the sautéed onions, reduce the heat to low, cover the pot and let cook for 20 to 25 minutes, until the kasha is tender and all the liquid has been absorbed.

Fluff with a fork and serve immediately.

Makes about 4 servings.

Extra Added Attraction

To turn this plain kasha dish into an Eastern European classic, toss the cooked kasha with an equal volume of cooked wide noodles or bow-tie pasta. A few sautéed mushrooms wouldn't hurt either.

Millet

Millet has been part of the human diet for millennia. It may even have been munched by dinosaurs, for all we know. It cooks quickly and it's delicious. It looks a little like couscous or quinoa, for which it can be substituted.

| 1 cup | 250 mL | hulled millet |
| 2½ cups | 625 mL | water (or stock, for added flavor) |

Place the millet in a large, dry skillet over medium-high heat. Cook, stirring constantly, until the millet grains turn golden, about 5 minutes. Remove from the heat.

In a medium saucepan with a tight-fitting lid, combine the toasted millet and water and bring to a boil over high heat. Reduce the heat to low, cover and let simmer until the grains are tender and the water has been absorbed, about 20 minutes.

Remove from the heat and let stand, covered, for 5 minutes.

Fluff with a fork and serve.

Makes 3 cups (750 mL).

Wild Rice

Technically speaking, wild rice is not really rice. But it looks like rice (sort of), cooks like rice (mostly), it's delicious (definitely) and it gets along nicely with brown rice and other grains. It's also rather expensive but very flavorful, so a little goes a long way. Toss a small amount of wild rice into a multigrain pilaf for a lavish touch or serve plain wild rice mixed with sautéed mushrooms or toasted pecans for all-out extravagance.

| 1 cup | 250 mL | wild rice |
| 4 cups | 1 L | water |

Pour the water into a medium saucepan with a tight-fitting lid. Bring it to a boil over high heat. Add the rice to the boiling water and give it a stir. Reduce the heat to the barest simmer and cover with the lid. Let cook for 35 minutes without peeking.

After 35 minutes, lift the lid and have a look. The water should be mostly absorbed, and the rice may be tender at this point. If not, replace the lid and let it cook for another 5 to 10 minutes, then check again. Cooking time for wild rice can vary quite a bit. (If the rice becomes tender before all the water has been absorbed, just drain off the excess water.) When the rice is done, remove the pan from the heat and let stand, covered, for 5 minutes, then fluff with a fork and serve.

Makes 4 to 5 cups (1 to 1.25 L).

Mexican Red Rice

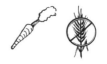

Make a double batch of this rice so that you'll have enough left over to stuff some Full-Meal Burritos (see page 159) later in the week. You'll be glad you did.

2 tbsp.	30 mL	olive oil or vegetable oil, divided
1		medium onion, chopped
1		clove garlic, minced or pressed
1 tsp.	5 mL	Mexican chili powder
1 cup	250 mL	diced tomatoes, canned or fresh (about 2 medium)
1 cup	250 mL	water or vegetable stock, homemade or store-bought (canned or from bouillon cubes or powder)
1 cup	250 mL	long-grain white rice
1 cup	250 mL	carrots or peas (or a mixture), diced, if desired
½ tsp.	2 mL	salt
¼ tsp.	1 mL	black pepper

Heat 1 tbsp. (15 mL) of the oil in a small saucepan over medium heat. Add the onion, garlic and chili powder and let cook for about 5 minutes, until the onions are softened.

Add the chopped tomatoes and cook, stirring, over medium-high heat for about 5 minutes, until the tomatoes have broken down into a sauce.

Dump the mixture into a blender or food processor along with the water or vegetable stock and blend until smooth.

Place the rice in a bowl and rinse thoroughly in several changes of cold water until the rinse water runs clear. Drain well.

Put the remaining 1 tbsp. (15 mL) of oil in a medium saucepan with a tight-fitting lid. Add the rinsed and drained rice and cook, stirring often, for 3 to 5 minutes, until the rice is glossy and beginning to turn yellow.

Add the blended tomato mixture, salt and pepper and bring it to a boil. Reduce the heat to low and cover the pot. Let simmer for 10 minutes.

Add the peas or carrots (or both), if you're using them, replace the cover and continue to cook for 5 to 10 minutes more, until the liquid is absorbed and the surface of the rice appears pitted with holes.

Remove from heat and let sit for 5 minutes before serving.

Makes 4 servings.

Easy Risotto

Most recipes for risotto insist that you stand at the stove, patiently stirring for what seems like an eternity. Who has that kind of time? Here's a recipe for risotto that frees you up to go set the table, take out the garbage or read your email while it cooks, all by itself, to creamy perfection.

2 tbsp.	30 mL	olive oil or vegetable oil
1 tbsp.	15 mL	butter (or use more oil, if you prefer)
1		medium onion, chopped
3 cups	750 mL	prepared vegetable of your choice (see page 169)
1½ cups	375 mL	Arborio rice
4 cups	1 L	vegetable stock, homemade or store-bought (canned or from bouillon cubes or powder)
½ tsp.	2 mL	salt
¼ tsp.	1 mL	black pepper
¼ cup	60 mL	grated Parmesan cheese, plus more to sprinkle at the table

In a medium saucepan with a tight-fitting lid, combine the oil and butter and place over medium heat. Add the onion and cook, stirring often, for 5 to 7 minutes, until softened and beginning to turn golden.

Add whichever vegetable you're using and cook, stirring, as described for each particular vegetable.

Add the rice to the saucepan and cook, stirring, for 1 or 2 minutes.

Add all the stock and bring to a boil, stirring to prevent the rice from sticking to the bottom of the pot. Reduce the heat to low, cover the pot with the lid and cook — no stirring or looking or any kind of fussing whatsoever — for 15 minutes.

After 15 miutes, remove the lid and stir in the Parmesan cheese, salt and pepper. The risotto should be creamy but not runny. If it seems too dry, you can add a bit of water or stock. The risotto will thicken as it cools.

Serve immediately with additional Parmesan cheese for sprinkling at the table.

Makes 4 servings.

Mushroom Risotto:

Slice 2 cups (500 mL) of mushrooms thinly, add at the appropriate step in the recipe and cook, stirring, for 5 to 7 minutes, until the mushrooms have released their juices and the liquid is almost completely evaporated.

Butternut Squash or Zucchini Risotto:

Peel a butternut squash and cut into ½-inch (1 cm) cubes (you'll need about 2 cups/500 mL squash for the recipe), or cut 2 small zucchinis into ½-inch (1 cm) cubes. Add at the appropriate step in the recipe and cook, stirring, for about 5 minutes. The squash will cook to tenderness as the risotto simmers.

Asparagus or Fresh Pea Risotto:

Trim 12 to 15 stalks of asparagus and cut into 1-inch (2 cm) lengths. If using peas, you'll need about 1½ cups (375 mL) fresh or frozen peas. (If using frozen peas, defrost before adding them to the pan.) Add the asparagus or peas to the risotto only after the rice has been cooking for 5 minutes.

Spinach Risotto:

Rinse and trim 1 (10 oz/284 g) bag of spinach (about 6 cups/1.5 L loose spinach leaves) and chop coarsely. Place in a covered saucepan and let the spinach cook in the water that clings to the leaves just until wilted. Drain. Add to the risotto only after the rice has been cooking for 10 minutes.

Cumin-Scented Yellow Rice

Fantastic with curry, excellent with chili, perfect with bean concoctions. Also very pretty.

1 tbsp.	15 mL	olive oil or vegetable oil
1		medium onion, chopped
1 tsp.	5 mL	whole cumin seeds
½ tsp.	2 mL	turmeric
½ tsp.	2 mL	salt
2 cups	500 mL	water
1 cup	250 mL	basmati or other long-grain white rice, well rinsed

Heat the oil in a medium saucepan over medium-low heat. Add the onion and cook, stirring often, for 5 to 7 minutes, until softened and beginning to turn golden.

Add the cumin seeds, turmeric and salt and continue cooking for 1 or 2 minutes, stirring constantly.

Add the water and rice, increase the heat to medium and bring to a boil. As soon as it boils, reduce the heat to low, cover the pot and let cook for about 15 minutes, until all the liquid has been absorbed and the rice is tender.

Makes 2 to 3 servings.

Bulgur Pilaf

Try this hearty pilaf instead of rice, pasta or couscous as an accompaniment to something saucy. It reheats well and will cheerfully wait around for the rest of dinner to be ready without going mushy.

2 tbsp.	30 mL	olive oil or vegetable oil
1 cup	250 mL	bulgur wheat
1		medium onion, chopped
2 cups	500 mL	vegetable stock, homemade or store-bought (canned or from bouillon cubes or powder)
2 tbsp.	30 mL	fresh parsley, chopped
½ tsp.	2 mL	salt
¼ tsp.	1 mL	black pepper

Heat the oil in a medium saucepan with a tight-fitting lid over medium heat. Add the bulgur and onion and cook, stirring, for 5 minutes, until the onion is softened.

Add the vegetable stock, parsley, salt and pepper and bring to a boil. Reduce the heat to low, cover the pot and let simmer until all the water is absorbed, about 20 to 25 minutes.

Fluff with a fork and serve.

Makes 4 servings.

Multigrain Pilaf

Serve this delicious pilaf as a side dish or bake it in a halved acorn or other small winter squash (see page 172). Substitute other cooked grains, like quinoa or millet, for the barley to make a gluten-free version, or toss in a can of drained beans to turn it into a main dish.

2 cups	500 mL	cooked brown rice
1 cup	250 mL	cooked wild rice
1 cup	250 mL	cooked barley
1 cup	250 mL	cooked corn kernels, fresh, frozen or canned
½ cup	125 mL	raisins or dried cranberries
2 tbsp.	30 mL	butter or non-dairy margarine
½ cup	125 mL	pecans, chopped
1 tsp.	5 mL	salt
¼ tsp.	1 mL	black pepper

Preheat the oven to 350°F (180°C). Grease an 8-cup (2 L) casserole dish with a lid.

In a large bowl, toss together the brown rice, wild rice, barley, corn kernels and raisins or cranberries.

Melt the butter or margarine in a small skillet over medium-low heat. Add the chopped pecans, and cook, stirring, until lightly toasted, about 5 minutes.

Add to the rice mixture along with salt and pepper and toss well. Transfer to the prepared casserole dish, cover and bake in the preheated oven for 20 to 25 minutes, until heated through.

Makes 4 to 6 servings.

Baked Stuffed Squash

Buy any small winter squash, like acorn squash, pepper squash, delicata squash or small buttercup squash. One medium squash will make 1 or 2 servings, depending on how fleshy the squash is.

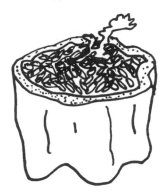

Remove the stem, cut each squash in half lengthwise and scoop out the seeds. Place the squash halves in a baking dish cut-side down, and pour a little water into the bottom to about ¼ inch (0.5 cm) deep. Bake at 425°F (220°C) for 20 minutes. Turn the squash halves over in the baking dish, brush the cut surfaces liberally with melted butter, olive oil or margarine, then:

- Fill the cavity of the squash halves with Multigrain Pilaf (see page 171); or
- stuff with your favorite chili and sprinkle with shredded cheese; or
- scoop in some leftover macaroni and cheese; or
- fill with any cooked vegetable mixture; or
- drizzle with maple syrup; or
- leave it empty.

Return to the oven and bake for 15 to 20 minutes, until the squash is completely tender when poked with a knife and the filling (if any) is heated through.

Basic Oven-Baked Polenta

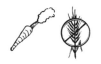

The traditional method for cooking polenta involves a lot of hanging around the stove and laborious stirring. But who says we have to be traditional? Try this recipe for perfect, creamy polenta, no laborious stirring required.

4 cups	1 L	water
1 cup	250 mL	cornmeal
1 tbsp.	15 mL	olive oil
1 tsp.	5 mL	salt

Preheat the oven to 350°F (180°C).

In a large ovenproof casserole or Dutch oven with a lid, combine the water, cornmeal, olive oil and salt. Cover the pot and place in the preheated oven. Bake, undisturbed, for 30 minutes.

Lift the lid, stir the polenta just until smooth, and then replace the lid and continue baking for an additional 20 to 25 minutes, until the polenta is soft and creamy.

Serve immediately, with something wonderfully saucy. Or use it to make Baked Polenta with Spinach and Cheese (page 134).

Makes 4 servings.

Sliceable Polenta

Pour the hot polenta onto a lightly greased baking sheet and chill until firm. This sheet of polenta can now be used in much the same way as lasagna noodles — layered with veggies, sauce and cheese and baked. Try it instead of regular noodles in the Irresistible Mushroom Lasagna (see page 110).

Very Happening Appetizer Recipe

Spread the soft polenta out in a greased 9 x 13-inch (23 x 33 cm) rectangular baking dish and chill until firm. Cut into squares or trapezoids, brush with a bit of olive oil and grill or broil until golden. Serve topped with a dab of goat cheese or pesto, some roasted peppers or whatever sounds like a good idea at the time.

Vegetables on the Side

Your Friend: The Potato

Where to start? Potatoes can be boiled, baked, steamed, roasted and fried. They can be mashed or cubed; they can be pureed in a soup; they can be hollowed out and stuffed. A perfect potato is a beautiful thing.

Fluffy Mashed Potatoes

Who doesn't love a creamy mound of mashed potatoes? Add butter or margarine, a splash of milk and you're done. Comfort food at its best.

4		medium potatoes, peeled and cut into chunks
½ cup	125 mL	milk, regular or non-dairy, heated until steaming
2 tbsp.	30 mL	butter or non-dairy margarine

First you'll have to cook the potatoes. You can boil them or steam them, whichever you prefer. To boil, place the potatoes in a saucepan with enough water to cover. Bring to a boil and let simmer until the potatoes are tender right through when poked with a fork. To steam, place potatoes in a steamer basket over boiling water. Cover the pot and steam until tender.

Either way, drain the potatoes thoroughly and return them to the pot in which they were cooked.

Add the milk and butter and mash with an official potato masher or with a fork until creamy, fluffy and perfect. Never use an electric mixer or food processor to mash potatoes — they become gummy when overbeaten. Besides, a few lumps in the finished product are proof that the potatoes are homemade.

Serve immediately with something saucy or use as a topping for Nearly Normal Shepherd's Pie (see page 132).

Makes 2 to 4 servings.

A Baked Potato

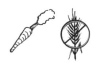

Nature's perfect food. Eat a plain baked potato with a sprinkle of salt and a dab of butter, and it will comfort you when you feel rotten. Muck it up with cheese and stuff, and it's a meal.

First of all, choose large potatoes without green spots or other blemishes. Any baking-type "russet" potato would be your obvious first choice, but any potato can be baked. Don't bother buying those individually foil-wrapped baking potatoes; loose potatoes are less expensive and you can actually see what you're getting. Besides, the foil isn't necessary for baking.

To Bake in a Regular Oven:
Preheat the oven to 400°F (200°C).
Thoroughly scrub as many potatoes as you want to bake and remove any sprouts. Poke them in several places with a fork. You can rub the skins all over with a bit of vegetable oil, if you like, or just leave them plain. Place potatoes directly on the rack in the preheated oven and bake for about 1 hour, until a potato feels soft when you gently squeeze it. Remove the potatoes from the oven, cut them in half and do whatever you like with them — they're now ready to eat. Plain or mucked-up (see below for suggestions).

To Bake in the Microwave:
Scrub no more than 4 potatoes as above and poke them in several places with a fork. Arrange them on a layer of paper towel, leaving space between them.

Microwave on high power: 1 potato for 4 minutes; 2 potatoes for 7 minutes; 3 potatoes for 9 minutes; 4 potatoes for 12 minutes.

Let stand for 3 or 4 minutes after baking and then have your way with them.

How to Muck up a Baked Potato:
- Cut the potatoes in half, scoop out the flesh and mash with a spoonful of sour cream and some chopped chives or green onion. Return the flesh to the shells, sprinkle with shredded cheddar and bake at 350°F (180°C) for 10 minutes, until heated through.
- Cut the potatoes in half, scoop out the flesh and mash with some roasted garlic (see page 27) and a drizzle of olive oil. Return the flesh to the shells, sprinkle with grated Parmesan cheese and bake at 350°F

(180°C) for 10 minutes, until heated through.

- Top baked potato halves with steamed broccoli and a sprinkle of cheddar cheese.
- Top baked potato halves with heated chili, a dollop of sour cream and a sprinkle of cheese.
- Bury potato halves in refried beans, salsa and sour cream.
- Top baked potato halves with scrambled eggs or scrambled tofu (see page 88) and a sprinkle of parsley.
- Slather baked potato halves with tomato sauce and sprinkle with pizza toppings and shredded mozzarella cheese. Bake at 350°F (180°C) for 10 minutes, until the cheese is melted.
- Scoop out the flesh and make Nacho-Stuffed Potato Shells (see page 36). Save the potato flesh for another use.

Un-Fried Potato Wedges

Crisp, brown and seriously addictive. Bet you can't eat just one.

4		large potatoes
2 tbsp.	30 mL	olive oil or vegetable oil
1 tsp.	5 mL	salt
¼ tsp.	1 mL	black pepper

Preheat the oven to 400°F (200°C). Grease a cookie sheet or baking pan large enough to hold all the potatoes without overlapping.

Scrub the potatoes well and cut into 6 or 8 lengthwise wedges, depending on the size of the potatoes. Smaller wedges will cook more quickly than chunky ones.

Place in a bowl, add the oil, salt and pepper and toss until all the potatoes are coated.

Dump onto the prepared pan and spread the potatoes out so that they're in a single layer.

Place in the oven and bake for 30 to 35 minutes, until the potatoes are beginning to brown on the bottom.

Flip the wedges around in the pan so that the browned side is up and continue to bake for an additional 20 minutes, until sizzling, crisp, nicely browned and irresistible.

Makes about 4 servings. (But probably not.)

Don't Leave Well Enough Alone

- Add ¼ tsp. (1 mL) cayenne pepper along with the salt and pepper.
- Add 2 minced cloves garlic and 1 tbsp. (15 mL) chopped fresh rosemary along with the salt and pepper.
- Double the amount of black pepper and add 2 tbsp. (30 mL) lemon juice along with the oil.
- Sprinkle the hot potato wedges with shredded cheddar or Parmesan cheese before eating.

Potato Kugel

Crisp and sizzling from the oven, this traditional potato casserole is usually served as a side dish, but it's substantial enough to be a main course. Your choice.

¼ cup	60 mL	vegetable oil
6		large potatoes, peeled
1		medium onion, finely chopped or grated
4		eggs, beaten
⅓ cup	75 mL	all-purpose flour
¼ cup	60 mL	fresh parsley, chopped, if desired
1 tsp.	5 mL	salt
¼ tsp.	1 mL	black pepper

Preheat the oven to 375°F (190°C). Pour the oil into a 9 x 13–inch (23 x 33 cm) rectangular baking dish. Set aside.

Using the shredding blade of a food processor or the large holes of a hand grater, grate the potatoes. Dump the grated potatoes into a colander and immediately run cold water over them — this prevents them from turning black (harmless but unappetizing).

Drain well, squeeze out as much water as possible and place in a large bowl. Add the onion, eggs, flour, parsley, salt and pepper and mix very well.

Place the baking dish containing the oil into the oven for about 5 minutes. (While this is happening, you can start cleaning up … Just a thought.)

Remove the baking dish from the oven and pour most of the hot oil into the potato mixture, leaving just enough in the baking dish to coat the bottom and sides. Stir the potato mixture well to incorporate the oil, and then dump into the baking dish — it should sizzle as it hits the pan — and pat it down in an even layer.

Place in the preheated oven and bake for about 1 hour, until the top is nicely browned. Serve immediately, cut into squares.

Makes about 12 servings.

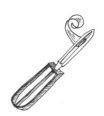

Just Plain Vegetables

Sometimes you just want a simple vegetable to go with your main dish. Here's a no-nonsense guide to preparing and cooking some of the most common ones. Just the basics here, seasonings are up to you.

Asparagus

Snap off the bottom of each stalk by gently bending the asparagus until it breaks. It should snap right at the point where the tender portion meets the tough portion. Rinse well and either cut into pieces or leave whole.

To cook: steam in a steamer basket over boiling water just until bright green or drizzle with a bit of olive oil and roast on a cookie sheet at 425°F (220°C) for 10 to 15 minutes, until sizzling.

Broccoli

Trim off the end of the stem and separate it from the florets. Cut the stem into chunks and the top into individual florets. Rinse well.

To cook: steam in a steamer basket over boiling water or simmer in water to cover until bright green and tender but still crisp.

Carrots

Scrub well and peel if you want. Cut into slices, cubes or sticks.

To cook: steam in a steamer basket over boiling water; or simmer in enough water or stock to cover; or sauté in oil or butter until tender but not mushy.

Cauliflower

Trim off any leaves and cut the head of cauliflower up into individual florets. Rinse well.

To cook: steam in a steamer basket over boiling water; or simmer in enough water to cover; or, best of all, toss with a bit of olive oil to coat, arrange in a single layer on a cookie sheet and roast at 425°F (220°C) for 20 to 40 minutes, until lightly browned.

Corn on the Cob

Peel off the husk and pull off the hairy bits.

To cook: steam in a steamer basket over boiling water; or boil in enough water to cover for at least 5 minutes but no more than 10 minutes; or cut from the cob and sauté with butter or oil and whatever else strikes your fancy.

Mushrooms

Rinse whole mushrooms and drain well. Trim stems and either leave whole or slice them or cut into chunks, depending on the size.

To cook: sauté in oil or butter until they release their liquid. Mushrooms play nicely with onions and garlic. And, of course, portobellos are delicious on the grill, but you already knew that.

Spinach

Pick over and remove any wilted leaves or non-spinach bits. Rinse well.

To cook: place rinsed spinach in a large pot — don't add any liquid — cover with a lid and cook over medium heat until the spinach is wilted. Done.

String Beans — Green, Yellow, Purple, Whatever

Green or yellow or purple or spotted — they're all good. Wash and snap off the stem end. Cut into pieces or leave whole.

To cook: steam in a steamer basket over boiling water or simmer in water until bright green and tender but still a little crisp.

Winter Squash — Butternut, Hubbard, Acorn, Delicate, Buttercup (and More)

Cut the squash in half and scoop out the seeds. Peel and cube or keep the halves intact.

To cook: cubed squash can be steamed in a steamer basket over boiling water or tossed with a little olive oil or butter and baked in a roasting pan at 400°F (200°C) until tender. Squash halves should be placed cut-side down on a cookie sheet or baking dish with just enough water to cover the bottom of the pan. Roast at 400°F (200°C) for 30 to 45 minutes, until tender. Turn halves over about halfway through the baking time to allow excess water to evaporate. Scoop out the flesh or, if small, serve on the half-shell.

Zucchini

Wash and cut crosswise into slices or dice into chunks.

To cook: sauté in a little olive oil or vegetable oil until tender. It's delicious combined with onions, garlic and tomatoes.

Four Quick Ways With Sweet Potatoes

- Bake them whole, like regular potatoes, until soft.
- Cut them into chunks, toss with olive oil, garlic, salt and pepper and roast on a cookie sheet at 425°F (220°C) until tender and caramelized.
- Bake, then peel and mash with maple syrup and butter or margarine.
- Peel, cube and steam until tender. Let cool and toss with Basic Vinaigrette Dressing.

Ratatouille

Ratatouille is a magical combination of zucchini, eggplant, tomatoes and peppers that manages to bring out the best in all the vegetables. You can, of course, serve it as a side dish, hot or at room temperature. Or you can serve it as a main course with pasta or rice or rolled into crepes.

2 tbsp.	30 mL	olive oil or vegetable oil
1		medium onion, chopped
4		cloves garlic, minced or pressed
2		medium green or red sweet peppers, diced
2		medium zucchini, cut into ½-inch (1 cm) cubes
1		medium eggplant, cut into ½-inch (1 cm) cubes
¼ cup	60 mL	fresh basil, chopped (or 1 tbsp./15 mL dried)
2 cups	500 mL	diced tomatoes, fresh (about 4 medium) or canned
½ tsp.	2 mL	salt
¼ tsp.	1 mL	black pepper

Heat the olive oil in a very large skillet or Dutch oven over medium heat. Add the onion and garlic and cook, stirring, for about 5 minutes, until softened.

Add the peppers, zucchini, eggplant and basil. Mix well and cook, stirring, for 10 minutes, until vegetables are almost tender.

Add the tomatoes, salt and pepper and cook for about 15 minutes, stirring occasionally, until the vegetables are tender and the flavors are blended. Serve hot or at room temperature.

Makes about 4 servings as a main dish or 8 servings as a side dish.

Sweet and Sour Red Cabbage with Apples

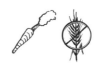

A perfect dish for a crisp day in fall. Add a Baked Stuffed Squash (see page 172) and some crusty whole-grain bread and it's a feast.

3 tbsp.	45 mL	olive oil or vegetable oil
2		medium onions, chopped
1		small head red cabbage, thinly sliced into shreds
2		apples, chopped (don't peel them)
½ cup	125 mL	red wine (any kind, even leftover yucky stuff is fine)
¼ cup	60 mL	apple cider (or other) vinegar
1 tbsp.	15 mL	granulated sugar
2 tsp.	10 mL	salt
½ cup	125 mL	red currant jelly or apple jelly

In a very large pot with a lid, heat the oil over medium heat. Add the onions and cook, stirring, for 5 minutes, until softened.

Add the shredded cabbage, reduce the heat slightly to medium-low and continue to cook for 10 to 15 minutes, until the cabbage is softened.

Stir in the apples, wine, vinegar, sugar and salt. Reduce the heat to low, cover the pot and let cook for for 1½ hours, stirring occasionally. (Go do something useful in the meantime, like read a book or eat cookies.) The cabbage should become very tender, but watch carefully so that it doesn't scorch on the bottom.

Stir in the red currant jelly, replace the cover and continue to simmer for another 15 to 20 minutes, until the flavors are blended.

Makes 8 to 10 very colorful servings.

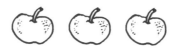

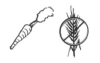

Baked-to-Death Tomatoes

Yes, the baking time is long, but it's not like you have to stand there and watch it or anything. Just slide the dish into the oven and go find something important to do. The tomatoes will bake, unattended, into a better, more tomatoey version of themselves. Amazing.

4		large tomatoes
2		cloves garlic, cut into slivers
4 tsp.	20 mL	olive oil
½ tsp.	2 mL	salt
¼ tsp.	1 mL	black pepper

Preheat the oven to 325°F (160°C).

Wash the tomatoes, remove the stem if there is one and cut each one in half crosswise through the "equator." Arrange the halves cut-side up in a single layer in a baking dish.

Stab garlic slivers into the cut side of the tomato halves, dividing them equally among the tomato halves.

Place in the oven and bake, uncovered, for 2 hours. Yes, really, t-w-o hours.

Open the oven, drizzle the tomato halves with olive oil and then sprinkle with salt and pepper.

Return to the oven and bake for 1 more hour. Yes. No kidding.

At the end of the baking time, remove the tomatoes from the oven and serve hot or let cool and serve at room temperature.

Makes 4 servings.

Tomato-Garlic Green Beans

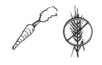

The green beans in this dish should be cooked until tender and squishy and infused with the flavors of the sauce. It's an especially good use for those green beans that have seen better days (you know, the ones at the back of your refrigerator).

2 tbsp.	30 mL	olive oil
1		large onion, chopped
2		cloves garlic, minced or pressed
2 cups	500 mL	diced tomatoes, fresh (about 2 medium) or canned
1 lb.	500 g	fresh green beans, cut into 1-inch (2 cm) pieces (about 4 cups/1 L)
1 tsp.	5 mL	crumbled dried oregano
1 tsp.	5 mL	salt
¼ tsp.	1 mL	black pepper

Heat the oil in a large skillet over medium heat. Add the onion and garlic and cook, stirring, for 8 to 10 minutes, until the onions are golden.

Add the tomatoes and bring to a simmer, stirring occasionally.

Now stir in the green beans, oregano, salt and pepper. Reduce the heat to low, cover and let simmer for about 30 minutes, stirring occasionally, until the beans are tender.

Makes 4 to 6 servings.

Oven-Roasted Vegetables

Feel free to vary this recipe to use whatever vegetables you happen to have. Just be sure to cut the veggies into big, chunky pieces so they don't cook too quickly — they need time to get all deliciously caramelized. You can serve these vegetables plain as a side dish, tossed with pasta or rice, or cooled to room temperature and drizzled with balsamic vinegar as a salad.

2		medium sweet potatoes, peeled and cut into 1-inch (2 cm) chunks
2		medium onions, peeled and cut into 1-inch (2 cm) chunks
1		large red sweet pepper, cored and cut into 1-inch (2 cm) squares
1		medium zucchini, cut into 1-inch (2 cm) chunks
½ lb.	250 g	mushrooms, whole or cut in half, if large (about 2½ cups/625 mL)
¼ cup	60 mL	olive oil
1 tbsp.	15 mL	fresh rosemary, chopped (or 1 tsp./5 mL dried)
½ tsp.	2 mL	salt
¼ tsp.	1 mL	black pepper

Preheat the oven to 425°F (220°C). Grease a large roasting pan (it should be big enough to hold all the vegetables in a single layer).

Place all the vegetables in a bowl and toss with the olive oil, rosemary, salt and pepper.

Spread the vegetables out in the prepared roasting pan. Don't crowd; they need room to brown properly.

Bake in the preheated oven for 40 to 45 minutes, tossing around occasionally, until all the vegetables are tender and well browned. Serve immediately or let cool and serve at room temperature.

Makes about 4 servings.

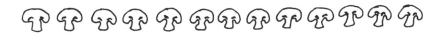

Shake and Bake Zucchini Sticks

Try these with some Tzatziki (see page 24) for dipping. Addictively excellent.

4 tbsp.	60 mL	vegetable oil, divided
4		medium zucchinis
½ cup	125 mL	bread crumbs
½ cup	125 mL	grated Parmesan cheese
½ tsp.	2 mL	garlic powder
½ tsp.	2 mL	salt
¼ tsp.	1 mL	black pepper
1		egg, beaten

Preheat the oven to 425°F (220°C). Pour 2 tbsp. (30 mL) of the vegetable oil onto a cookie sheet and spread it to coat the bottom evenly.

Trim the stem and blossom ends off the zucchini and cut them into sticks approximately ½ inch (1 cm) thick and 3 inches (8 cm) long.

In a small bowl, mix together the bread crumbs, Parmesan cheese, garlic powder, salt and pepper. Dump this mixture into a clean plastic bag.

Working with about 3 or 4 zucchini sticks at a time, first dip them into the beaten egg, then fish them out (letting the excess egg drip back into the bowl) and toss them into the bag with the bread crumb mixture. Shake to coat. Remove coated zukes from the bag and arrange them on the baking sheet. Repeat until you have used up all the zucchini sticks or crumbs or (ideally) both.

Drizzle the remaining 2 tbsp. (30 mL) of oil over the breaded zucchini sticks, place the pan in the preheated oven and bake for 15 to 20 minutes, turning them over about halfway through the baking time. They should be nicely browned and sizzling. Serve immediately.

Makes about 4 servings.

Spicy Sautéed Corn

There's only so much plain corn on the cob you can eat before you begin to feel the urge to mess with it. A little garlic, a dash of cayenne and a splodge of cream or milk will definitely do the trick.

4		cobs fresh corn
2 tbsp.	30 mL	butter or non-dairy margarine
2		cloves garlic, minced or pressed
½ tsp.	2 mL	salt
¼ tsp.	1 mL	cayenne pepper, or more (if you want lots of heat)
½ cup	125 mL	milk, regular or non-dairy (or, to be truly decadent, cream)

With a sharp knife, cut the corn kernels off the cobs, scraping the cobs to remove as much of the pulp as possible. Set the kernels aside.

Melt the butter in a large skillet, add the corn kernels, garlic, salt and cayenne and cook, stirring, for 5 to 6 minutes, until the corn is tender but still crisp.

Add the milk or cream and let simmer for another 3 to 4 minutes, until the sauce is creamy and the corn is tender. Serve immediately, plain or spooned over rice.

Makes 2 to 3 servings.

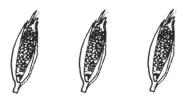

8. Baked Stuff

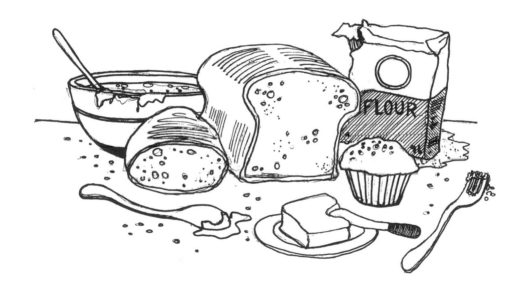

Ultra-Quick All-Purpose Yeast Dough

Who has time to hang around for ages waiting for dough to rise? Not you. This easy recipe will let you whip up a pizza crust, a slab of focaccia or a fabulous loaf of bread and still have a life. The secret is something called "quick-rise" instant yeast (available everywhere, alongside regular yeast granules), which does the job in half the time of the ordinary kind.

3½ cups	875 mL	all-purpose flour, divided
1 envelope		quick-rise instant yeast (or 2¼ tsp./11 mL granules)
1 tsp.	5 mL	salt
1 cup	250 mL	hot tap water
2 tbsp.	30 mL	olive oil or vegetable oil, plus additional to oil the bowl

In a large bowl, stir together 2 cups (500 mL) of the flour, the yeast and salt. Add the hot water and oil and stir until the mixture is smooth (it will be sticky and gooey, which is fine).

Now add ½ cup of the remaining flour and mix it in with a sturdy spoon. Keep adding flour, ½ cup (125 mL) at a time, and mixing it in until the mixture starts to become hard to stir.

At this point, dump about ½ cup (125 mL) of flour onto your counter or table (you will have some left after mixing the dough), and spread it around a bit to form a well-floured kneading area. Turn the sticky lump of dough out onto this floured surface and sprinkle the top of the lump with a little flour so it won't stick to your hands. Begin kneading the dough by hand, adding only as much of the total amount of flour as is necessary to keep it from sticking to your hands (or the table). Continue to knead for at least 8 to 10 minutes, until the dough is no longer sticky and its surface is smooth and pliable (it will feel like your earlobe — really). You may not use the entire amount of flour, which is okay.

Lightly oil a large bowl. Transfer the kneaded dough to the bowl, turning it over so that all sides of the blob are oiled.

Cover the bowl with plastic wrap and place in a warmish spot for the dough to rise until it's doubled in size (you don't need to get out the calipers, just eyeball it). It can take anywhere from 20 to 40 minutes for the dough to rise, depending on complex cosmic factors. Be patient.

When the dough has doubled, punch it down to deflate it completely (fun!) then knead it a few times until smooth. Let the dough rest for 5 minutes before using it to make pizza (see page 144) or focaccia (see page 192).

Makes enough dough to make two 12-inch (30 cm) pizzas or two pans of foccaccia.

Raising Yeast Dough

So the recipe tells you to place your dough in a warm spot to rise. But what, exactly, does that mean? How warm? Where? Is the oven too warm? The broom closet not warm enough? Here are a few suggestions:

- Place a large pan of hot tap water on the bottom rack or floor of your oven. Place the bowl of dough on the rack directly above it. Do not turn the oven on! The heat and moisture from the hot water will warm the oven just enough and keep the surface of the dough from drying out. A perfect cozy spot.
- Place a large measuring cup filled with water into the microwave. Nuke until the water boils. Now put your bowl of dough into the microwave, leaving the measuring cup in there with it. Close the door. Warm and humid. Ideal.
- Cover your bowl of dough with plastic wrap and place it on top of your refrigerator. For many refrigerators, but not all, this is a warm spot. The plastic wrap will keep the surface of the dough from drying out.
- Cover the bowl of dough with plastic wrap and place in the cupboard directly above your stove. If you've been cooking, it will be a warm place for the dough to rise.

Honey Wheat Bread

If you've never made an actual loaf of bread before, try this simple classic.

5 cups	1.25 L	all-purpose white flour, divided
2 cups	500 mL	whole-wheat flour
2 envelopes		quick-rise instant yeast (or 4½ tsp./22 mL granules)
2 tsp.	10 mL	salt
2 cups	500 mL	milk, regular or non-dairy
½ cup	125 mL	water
½ cup	125 mL	honey
2 tbsp.	30 mL	vegetable oil, plus additional to oil the bowl

In a very large bowl, stir together 4 cups (1 L) of the all-purpose white flour, all the whole-wheat flour, the yeast and the salt.

In a small saucepan, combine the milk, water, honey and vegetable oil and place over medium heat until the mixture is just hot to the touch but not boiling, around 110°F to 120°F (225°C to 250°C).

Add the milk mixture to the flour mixture and mix in with a sturdy spoon. Add ½ of the remaining flour and mix it in. Keep adding flour ½ cup (125 mL) at a time and mixing it in until the mixture becomes too hard to stir.

Now sprinkle about ½ cup (125 mL) of the remaining white flour on your table or counter and spread it around to form a well-floured kneading area. Dump the sticky dough out onto this surface. Sprinkle the dough with a bit more of the flour and begin to knead. Keep kneading the dough, sprinkling it with flour, for 8 to 10 minutes, until it no longer sticks to your hands or the counter. Your dough should be smooth and feel like your earlobe when you pinch it. You may not use the entire amount of flour, which is okay.

Lightly oil a large bowl. Place the blob of dough into the bowl and turn it over to grease all sides. Cover with plastic wrap and place in a warm spot to rise until doubled in size, about 30 to 40 minutes.

Preheat the oven to 375°F (190°C). Grease two 9 x 5 x 3–inch (23 x 12 x 7 cm) loaf pans.

Remove the unsuspecting dough from wherever it's been rising and punch your fist into it to deflate it.

Knead the dough a couple of times, and then divide it into two equal pieces. Form each one into a loaf shape and place them into the prepared pans. Cover loosely with plastic wrap or a clean dish towel, place in a warm spot and let rise again, for about 30 minutes, until not quite double in size.

Place the loaves in the preheated oven and bake for 30 to 40 minutes, until they're golden brown on top and sound hollow when you tap on them. If you're not quite sure, let bake for 5 minutes more and check again.

Remove your perfectly gorgeous bread from the pans and, for heaven's sake, have the decency to let them cool for a least a few minutes before devouring. Did you do that? Wow.

Makes 2 loaves.

Oatmeal Raisin Bread

The essential breakfast loaf. Awesome toasted.

5 to 6 cups	1.25 to 1.5 L	all-purpose white flour, divided
2½ cups	625 mL	quick-cooking (not instant) rolled oats, plus more for sprinkling
¼ cup	60 mL	brown sugar
2 envelopes		quick-rise instant yeast (or 4½ tsp./22 mL granules)
2 tsp.	10 mL	salt
1½ cups	375 mL	water
1¼ cups	310 mL	milk, regular or non-dairy
¼ cup	60 mL	vegetable oil
½ cup	125 mL	raisins, soaked in boiling water and drained

In a very large bowl, stir together 3 cups (750 mL) of the all-purpose white flour, all the oats, the brown sugar, yeast and salt.

In a small saucepan, combine the water, milk and oil and heat until steaming but not boiling, around 110°F to 120°F (225°C–250°C).

Add the liquid to the flour mixture and stir until everything is well combined. Now, add ½ cup of the remaining white flour and mix it in. Keep adding flour ½ cup (125 mL) at a time until the dough becomes too stiff to stir in the bowl. It will still be pretty sticky at this point.

Now sprinkle a generous amount of the remaining white flour onto your table or counter to form a well-floured kneading area. Turn the sticky dough out onto this surface and sprinkle the surface of the dough with a bit more of flour. Begin to knead. Keep kneading the dough, sprinkling it with flour, for 8 to 10 minutes, until it no longer sticks to your hands or the counter and is fairly smooth. (The oats will make it a little bumpy.)

Lightly oil a large bowl. Place the dough in the bowl and turn the dough over to grease all sides. Cover with plastic wrap and place in a warm spot to rise until it's doubled in size, about 30 to 40 minutes.

Preheat the oven to 375°F (190°C). Grease two 9 x 5 x 3–inch (23 x 12 x 7 cm) loaf pans.

Uncover the bowl of dough and punch your fist into the dough to deflate it. Knead the dough a couple of times and — ta da! — it's time to make your loaves. Cut the dough in half, shape it into two loaves and place the loaves in the prepared pans. Lightly cover the loaves with plastic wrap or a clean dish towel and let them rise again in a warm spot until they're not quite doubled in size, about 20 to 30 minutes.

Brush the tops of the loaves with a little warm water or milk, sprinkle with a few flakes of rolled oats and bake for 35 to 45 minutes, until deep golden brown.

Remove from the pans and let cool for at least a few minutes before devouring.

Makes 2 gorgeous loaves.

Fabulous Focaccia

You can load your focaccia down with toppings or just leave it simple. Whatever you do, it'll be great.

¼ cup	60 mL	olive oil or vegetable oil
2		onions, sliced
4		cloves garlic, minced or pressed
1 recipe		Ultra-Quick All-Purpose Yeast Dough (see page 188)
¼ cup	60 mL	grated Parmesan cheese, if desired
1 tsp.	5 mL	crumbled dried rosemary or oregano
½ tsp.	2 mL	salt
¼ tsp.	1 mL	black pepper

Grease two cookie sheets or pizza pans and sprinkle them with cornmeal.

Heat the oil in a large skillet over medium heat. Add the onions and garlic and cook, stirring occasionally, for 5 to 7 minutes, until softened. Set aside to cool for a few minutes.

Divide the prepared dough into two pieces. Working with one piece at a time, flatten the dough out by hand or with a rolling pin to an 8-inch (20 cm) circle that's about ½-inch (1 cm) thick. Place on the

A Simple Focaccia

Instead of the whole onion business, just make little indentations all over the surface of the risen dough rounds with your fingertips and brush the dough liberally with olive oil. Sprinkle with a bit of coarse salt, some pepper and a little crumbled rosemary. Bake as for Fabulous Focaccia.

prepared pan. Repeat with the other piece of dough.

Spoon the onion mixture onto the two rounds of dough, dividing the mixture equally and spreading it out almost to the edges.

Sprinkle with grated Parmesan, rosemary or oregano, salt and pepper. Place the dough rounds in a warm place to rise, lightly covered with plastic wrap or a clean dish towel for 20 to 30 minutes, until a little puffy.

Preheat the oven to 375°F (190°C).

Place the breads in the oven and bake for 20 to 25 minutes, until the bottom of the focaccias are lightly browned and the top crust is golden. Eat while still warm if possible.

Makes two 10-inch (30 cm) breads.

Jalapeño Corn Bread

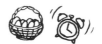

Is there a more perfect accompaniment to a bowl of chili? We think not.

1½ cups	375 mL	all-purpose white flour
1 cup	250 mL	yellow cornmeal
2 tbsp.	30 mL	granulated sugar
2 tbsp.	30 mL	baking powder
1 tsp.	5 mL	salt
1⅓ cups	325 mL	milk, regular or non-dairy
1		egg
¼ cup	60 mL	vegetable oil
¼ cup	60 mL	fresh or canned jalapeño peppers, chopped
½ tsp.	2 mL	crushed red pepper flakes, if desired

Preheat the oven to 350°F (180°C). Grease an 8-inch (20 cm) square baking pan.

Put the flour, cornmeal, sugar, baking powder and salt in a large bowl and stir to mix.

In a small bowl, whisk together the milk, egg and oil. Pour the milk mixture into the flour mixture and stir until combined. A few lumps are okay — resist the temptation to overbeat. Fold in the chopped jalapeño peppers and red pepper flakes (if you're using them).

Pour the batter into the prepared baking pan, smooshing the top so that it's smooth.

Place in the preheated oven and bake for 20 to 25 minutes, until a toothpick poked into the middle comes out clean.

Let cool for a few minutes before cutting into squares and serve warm.

Makes about 9 big hunks.

Biscuit Mix

Here's a homemade version of that pantry staple — but way better than anything you can buy. Made with butter, not hydrogenated shortening, this tastes delicious and has none of that nasty trans-fat stuff. It can be used as a straight substitute in any recipe that calls for commercial biscuit mix and will keep, refrigerated, for a long time.

9 cups	2.25 L	all-purpose white flour (or 4½ cups/1125 mL each white and whole-wheat flour)
¼ cup	60 mL	baking powder
2 tsp.	10 mL	salt
2 tsp.	10 mL	cream of tartar
1 tsp.	5 mL	baking soda
1 lb.	500 g	cold butter

In a large bowl, stir together the flour, baking powder, salt, cream of tartar and baking soda until well mixed.

Using a pastry blender, cut the butter into the flour mixture until the mixture resembles coarse cornmeal. This can also be done in 2 or 3 batches in a food processor; just make sure you divide the ingredients equally and don't overprocess the mixture. It should remain mealy.

Store the mixture in the refrigerator or freezer in a tightly covered container. Use in any recipe that calls for commercial biscuit mix.

Makes about 10 cups (2.5 L).

Biscuits from Scratch (or Not)

Don't bother trying to resist.

From scratch:

2 cups	500 mL	all-purpose white flour (or 1 cup/250 mL each all-purpose white and whole-wheat)
4 tsp.	20 mL	baking powder
1 tbsp.	15 mL	granulated sugar (if desired — for a sweet biscuit)
½ tsp.	2 mL	salt
½ cup	125 mL	butter or non-dairy margarine
¾ cup	175 mL	milk, regular or non-dairy

From mix:

2 cups	500 mL	biscuit mix, homemade (see page 194) or store-bought
½ cup	125 mL	milk, regular or non-dairy

Preheat the oven to 425°F (220°C).

If you are making your biscuits from scratch, stir together the flour, baking powder, sugar (if using) and salt in a mixing bowl. With a pastry blender or two knives, cut in the butter or margarine until the mixture is crumbly and resembles dry oatmeal. Add the milk, stirring until the mixture is combined and can be gathered together into a ball of dough.

If you are using biscuit mix, stir together the mix with the milk just until it forms a soft dough.

For both methods, on a lightly floured surface, gently roll or pat the dough out to about ½ inch (1 cm) thick.

Cut biscuits out with a 2-inch (5 cm) round cookie cutter (or a drinking glass dipped in flour). Place the biscuits on an ungreased cookie sheet and bake in the preheated oven for 10 to 12 minutes, until lightly browned.

If you're not in the mood to mess around or if, for some reason, your dough is too soft to roll out, simply scoop spoonfuls of dough out onto an ungreased cookie sheet and bake as above.

Makes 10 to 12 biscuits.

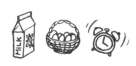

Parmesan Onion Bread

A great savory bread for eating as a snack — even better to serve alongside a bowl of soup.

2 cups	500 mL	biscuit mix, homemade (see page 194) or store-bought
¾ cup	175 mL	milk
1		small onion, finely chopped
½ cup	125 mL	grated Parmesan cheese
½ cup	125 mL	mayonnaise
1 tbsp.	15 mL	jalapeño pepper, finely chopped, if desired (but good)

Preheat the oven to 400°F (200°C). Grease an 8- or 9-inch (20 or 23 cm) square baking pan.

In a bowl, stir together the biscuit mix and the milk, and combine to make a soft dough.

By hand, squash the dough evenly into the prepared baking pan, covering the entire bottom.

In another bowl, stir together the onion, Parmesan cheese, mayonnaise and jalapeño pepper (if using). Spread this stuff evenly over the dough in the pan.

Place in the preheated oven and bake for 18 to 20 minutes, until browned on the edges.

Cut into squares and serve while still warm.

Makes 6 to 8 servings.

Ridiculously Easy Cheese Quick Bread

This quick bread doesn't need kneading or rising. Whatever you don't eat right away can be used to make a super sandwich.

2 cups	500 mL	all-purpose flour (or 1 cup/250 mL each white and whole-wheat)
4 tsp.	20 mL	baking powder
1 tbsp.	15 mL	granulated sugar
½ tsp.	2 mL	dry mustard powder
½ tsp.	2 mL	salt
1¼ cups	310 mL	shredded cheese (cheddar, Monterey Jack, Swiss)
1		egg
1 cup	250 mL	milk, regular or non-dairy
2 tbsp.	30 mL	vegetable oil

Preheat the oven to 375°F (190°C). Grease a 9 x 5 x 3–inch (23 x 12 x 7 cm) loaf pan.

In a large bowl, stir together the flour, baking powder, sugar, mustard powder, salt and cheese.

In a small bowl, whisk together the egg, milk and oil.

All at once, pour the egg mixture into the flour mixture and stir just until all of the ingredients are moistened. The batter will be lumpy, but that's okay.

Spoon batter into the prepared loaf pan and bake for 45 to 50 minutes, until the top is beginning to brown lightly.

Allow the bread to cool in the pan for about 10 minutes before removing it from the pan to continue cooling. Eat warm or at room temperature, but it's really best when it's warm.

Makes 1 ridiculously easy loaf.

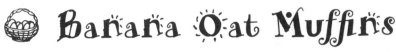# Banana Oat Muffins

These muffins are a dignified demise for those poor black bananas that have been festering on the counter all week.

¾ cup	175 mL	all-purpose flour
½ cup	125 mL	quick-cooking (not instant) rolled oats
½ cup	125 mL	granulated sugar
1 tsp.	5 mL	baking soda
½ tsp.	2 mL	baking powder
½ cup	125 mL	vegetable oil
2		medium-sized ripe bananas
2		eggs

Preheat the oven to 375°F (190°C). Grease a 12-compartment muffin pan.

In a large bowl, stir together the flour, oats, sugar, baking soda and baking powder.

In the container of a blender or food processor (or with a hand-held blender), blend together the oil, bananas and eggs until smooth.

Pour the banana mixture into the flour mixture and stir just until combined.

Spoon the batter into the prepared muffin pan, filling the cups almost to the top. (There may not be enough batter to fill all of the compartments.)

Place in the preheated oven and bake for 25 to 30 minutes, until a toothpick poked into the middle of a muffin comes out clean.

Serve the muffins warm or at room temperature.

Makes about 9.

Fill-er-up

If you're making muffins and don't have enough batter to fill all of the compartments, pour a little water into the empty sections before baking. It helps the muffins bake more evenly and will make the pan easier to wash afterward.

Carrot Apple Muffins

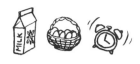

Not too sweet, not too cakey, these muffins are a very cheery way to start your morning.

2		eggs
½ cup	125 mL	granulated sugar
½ cup	125 mL	plain yogurt
¼ cup	60 mL	vegetable oil
1 cup	250 mL	all-purpose flour (or ½ cup/125 mL each white and whole-wheat)
1 tsp.	5 mL	baking soda
½ tsp.	2 mL	cinnamon
¾ cup	175 mL	carrot (about 1 medium carrot), shredded scrubbed
¾ cup	175 mL	apple (about 1 medium apple), shredded peeled and cored
½ cup	125 mL	walnuts, chopped

Preheat the oven to 375°F (190°F). Grease a 12-compartment muffin pan.

In a medium bowl, whisk together the eggs, sugar, yogurt and vegetable oil until very well mixed.

In a small bowl, stir together the flour, baking soda and cinnamon.

Add the flour mixture to the egg mixture and stir until smooth. Add the shredded carrot, apple and nuts and stir until just combined.

Spoon the batter into the prepared muffin pan, filling the cups almost to the top.

Bake in the preheated oven for 20 to 25 minutes, until a toothpick poked into the middle of a muffin comes out clean.

Serve warm or at room temperature.

Makes about 9 muffins.

9. Just Desserts

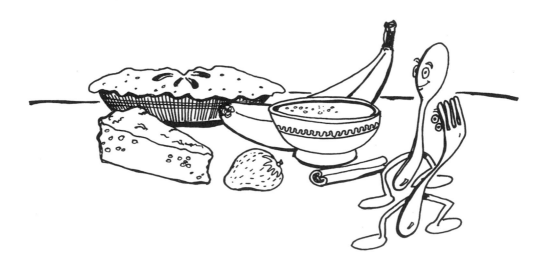

Vegetarians and vegans deserve a great dessert as much as anyone. All the recipes in this section are vegan-friendly — no eggs are required and non-dairy substitutions are no problem. So go ahead, indulge. You've earned it.

Amazing Eggless Dairy-Free Chocolate Cake

Just because you don't use eggs or dairy doesn't mean you shouldn't have your chocolate cake (and eat it too). This one is so absolutely delicious that no one will believe how easy it is to make.

1½ cups	375 mL	all-purpose white flour
1 cup	250 mL	granulated sugar
¼ cup	60 mL	unsweetened cocoa powder
1 tsp.	5 mL	baking soda
1 cup	250 mL	water
⅓ cup	75 mL	vegetable oil
1 tsp.	5 mL	white vinegar
1 tsp.	5 mL	vanilla extract

Preheat the oven to 350°F (180°C). Grease an 8-inch (20 cm) square pan.

In a medium bowl, stir together the flour, sugar, cocoa powder and baking soda until evenly combined.

All at once, add the water, oil, vinegar and vanilla. Quickly stir until well mixed, and then dump the batter into the prepared baking pan.

Place in the oven and bake for 30 to 35 minutes, until a toothpick poked into the center of the cake comes out clean. Let cool completely before frosting (if desired).

Now what could possibly be easier?

Makes one 8-inch (20 cm) square cake.

Note:

This recipe can be doubled to make a two-layer chocolate cake. Bake the batter in two well-greased 9-inch (23 cm) round pans. Baking time remains the same.

Amazing Eggless Dairy-Free Vanilla Cake

Here's the vanilla counterpart to the chocolate cake recipe because vegans cannot live by chocolate alone. Although it would be nice.

1½ cups	375 mL	all-purpose flour
¾ cup	175 mL	granulated sugar
1 tbsp.	15 mL	baking powder
1 cup	250 mL	milk, regular or non-dairy
⅓ cup	75 mL	vegetable oil
1 tsp.	5 mL	vanilla extract

Preheat the oven to 350°F (180°C). Grease an 8-inch (20 cm) square baking pan.

In a medium bowl, stir together the flour, sugar and baking powder until well mixed.

All at once, add the milk, vegetable oil and vanilla. Stir just until the batter is smooth, and then dump into the prepared baking pan.

Place in the preheated oven and bake for 30 to 35 minutes, until a toothpick poked into the middle of the cake comes out clean and it is lightly browned on top.

Cool completely before slathering it with icing (if that's what you plan to do) or burying it under some lovely fresh berries.

Makes one 8-inch (20 cm) square cake.

Note:

This recipe can be doubled to make a two-layer vanilla cake. Bake the batter in two well-greased 9-inch (23 cm) round pans. Baking time remains the same.

Two Fabulous Frostings

Both of these frostings can be made with either butter or non-dairy margarine. When shopping for non-dairy margarine, look for the word "pareve" on the package, which tells you that the product contains no dairy ingredients and can be eaten by vegans or anyone else who avoids dairy.

Chocolate Frosting

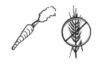

1 cup	250 mL	softened butter or non-dairy margarine
2 cups	500 mL	confectioner's sugar (powdered icing sugar)
½ cup	125 mL	unsweetened cocoa powder
½ tsp.	2 mL	vanilla extract
1 tbsp.	15 mL	milk, regular or non-dairy, if needed

In a food processor, or in a large bowl and using an electric mixer, beat the butter or margarine until smooth and creamy.

Add the sugar, cocoa and vanilla and beat until smooth and fluffy.

Add the milk, drop by drop, only if the frosting seems too stiff. (You may not need to use it at all.)

Makes enough frosting for a 9-inch (23 cm) two-layer cake.

Vanilla Frosting

1 cup	250 mL	softened butter or non-dairy margarine
1 tsp.	5 mL	vanilla extract
3 cups	750 mL	confectioner's sugar (powdered icing sugar)
1 tbsp.	15 mL	milk, regular or non-dairy, if needed

In a food processor, or in a large bowl and using an electric mixer, beat the butter or margarine until very smooth and creamy.

Add the sugar and vanilla and continue beating until smooth and fluffy.

Add the milk, drop by drop, only if the frosting seems too stiff. (You may not need to use it at all.)

Makes enough frosting for a 9-inch (23 cm) two-layer cake.

Fruit Crumble

Use whatever fruit is in season to make a wonderful fruit crumble. You can even use frozen fruit or make it with a mixture of wrinkly odds and ends.

6 cups	1.5 L	prepared fruit (see fruit ideas below)
½ cup	125 mL	granulated sugar
2 tbsp.	30 mL	cornstarch
1 cup	250 mL	all-purpose white or whole-wheat flour
½ cup	125 mL	butter or non-dairy margarine
½ cup	125 mL	brown sugar
½ tsp.	2 mL	cinnamon, if desired (depending on the fruit)

Preheat the oven to 375°F (190°C). Grease an 8- or 9-inch (20 or 23 cm) square baking dish.

In a large bowl, toss the fruit, whatever you're using, with the granulated sugar and cornstarch. (You may want to adjust the amount of sugar, depending on the sweetness of the fruit. Go ahead, it'll turn out fine anyway.) Dump into the prepared baking dish.

In a food processor, or in a bowl and using a fork or pastry blender, combine the flour, butter or margarine, brown sugar and cinnamon (if using). Mix and mash until the mixture is a crumbly, moist mess.

Sprinkle the crumbles evenly over the top of the fruit in the baking dish.

Place in the oven and bake for 35 to 45 minutes, until the fruit is bubbly and tender and the topping is crisp and golden.

Serve warm or at room temperature with regular or non-dairy ice cream, frozen yogurt or whipped cream. Killer.

Makes 6 to 8 servings.

Fruit ideas:

Apples or pears – peeled, cored and sliced
Peaches – peeled, pitted and sliced
Rhubarb – cut into chunks
Blueberries, strawberries or raspberries
Plums – pitted and quartered
Tutti-frutti – just a fancy way of saying a little of whatever you've got!

Ye Olde Creamy Rice Pudding

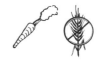

An old-fashioned dessert, it's best eaten on a rainy evening in front of the TV. But also suitable for sunny afternoons with a good book.

2 cups	500 mL	water
1 cup	250 ml	Arborio rice (or other short-grain white rice)
1½ cups	375 mL	milk, regular or non-dairy
½ cup	125 mL	granulated sugar
1 tsp.	5 mL	vanilla extract
½ cup	125 mL	raisins, if desired
		cinnamon, for sprinkling

In a medium saucepan, combine the water and rice and bring to a boil over medium heat.

Reduce the heat to low, cover the pot and let cook until all the water has been absorbed and the rice is tender, about 15 minutes.

Uncover the pot, stir in the milk, sugar and vanilla and continue to cook, stirring often, for 10 to 15 minutes, until creamy and thickened. If you're using the raisins, stir them in after the pudding has been cooking for about 5 minutes.

Cool the pudding then chill it in the refrigerator. The pudding will thicken as it cools, so you may want to stir in a bit of additional milk before spooning into dishes, sprinkling with cinnamon and serving.

Makes about 4 servings.

Fantastic Fruit Sorbet

This sorbet can be made with almost any kind of fruit — like strawberries, raspberries, mangoes, peaches, melons, pineapple — fresh, frozen or canned. It really is fantastic.

1 cup	250 mL	water
½ cup	125 mL	granulated sugar
3 cups	750 mL	fruit (see sidebar)
2 tbsp.	30 mL	lemon juice

Sorbet-Worthy Fruit Possibilities

Berries — any kind. Rinse and drain. Fresh peaches or **Nectarines** — peel, remove pit and cut flesh into chunks. **Mangoes** — peel, remove pit and cut flesh into chunks. **Melons** — cut in half, scoop out the seeds, peel the flesh and cut into chunks. **Pineapple** — peel and cut into chunks.

In a small saucepan, bring the water and sugar to a boil over medium-high heat, stirring only until the sugar is dissolved. Let this mixture cook for exactly 5 minutes (timing from the minute it comes to a boil), and then remove it from heat and let cool to room temperature.

Prepare whatever fruit you're using by peeling, pitting and cutting it into cubes. If it's frozen, defrost it (save the juice). Berries can be left whole.

Place your prepared fruit in the container of a food processor or blender and blend until pureed, like baby food.

Add the sugar syrup to the fruit puree and mix well.

Pour into an 8-inch (20 cm) square metal baking pan and place in the freezer. Let freeze until solid, at least 3 to 4 hours.

Remove the pan from the freezer and scoop the frozen fruit mixture into the container of a food processor. Process until smooth and creamy, scraping down the sides of the bowl once or twice so that it blends evenly.

Spoon the sorbet into a bowl or other container and return it to the freezer for about 30 minutes or until you're ready to serve it.

Makes 4 servings.

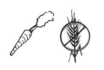

Frozen Chocolate Bananasicles

Feed your inner kid with this easy but irresistible treat.

1 cup	250 mL	chocolate chips
2		large bananas
½ cup	125 mL	chopped peanuts or shredded coconut

Melt the chocolate chips in a small saucepan set into another saucepan filled with boiling water (or in a double boiler), stirring until smooth.

Peel bananas and cut them in half crosswise.

Insert wooden popsicle sticks (or something similar) into the cut ends of each piece of banana.

Dip the bananas into melted chocolate to coat completely. Roll in chopped peanuts or coconut.

Place the bananas on a waxed-paper lined baking sheet and freeze for several hours, until firm.

Whatever you don't eat right away should be wrapped in plastic wrap and stored in the freezer for future munching.

Makes 4 bananasicles.

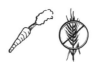

Fruit Compote

You had a good reason for buying that basket of peaches, apples, pears, whatever. Only now you can't remember what it was. And — yikes — they're all-too-quickly decomposing on your counter. Quick! Make some compote!

6 cups	1.5 L	fruit
½ cup	125 mL	granulated sugar, or less (to taste)
1		cinnamon stick

Rummage through your fruit and cut out any squishy or rotten parts. Prepare it by peeling, coring, pitting and cutting the flesh into slices or chunks, whatever is appropriate for the fruit you have. You can use apples, peaches, plums, pears, cherries, nectarines — any mixture of fruit will do.

Dump the fruit into a medium saucepan along with the sugar and cinnamon. Let sit at room temperature for about 30 minutes, until the juices are drawn out, then bring to a boil over medium-low heat. Cook, stirring gently — don't mash up the fruit — for about 10 minutes, until everything is tender.

Cool to room temperature then chill.

Serve compote in a pretty dish or spoon over some plain cake. A dollop of whipped cream or yogurt? Why not?

Makes about 6 servings.

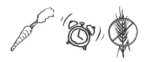

Peach and Banana Flambé

There's nothing like a flaming dessert to wake up your dinner guests. Make sure you prepare this in view of everyone to take full advantage of the spectacle.

3		medium bananas
2		large peaches
1 tbsp.	15 mL	lemon juice
¼ cup	60 mL	butter or non-dairy margarine
⅔ cup	150 mL	brown sugar
¼ cup	60 mL	light rum, brandy or other liqueur

Peel the bananas and cut, crosswise, into diagonal slices about ½ inch (1 cm) thick.

Peel the peaches, remove the pits and slice thickly.

Place the bananas and peaches in a bowl and toss with lemon juice.

In a large skillet, melt the butter or margarine over medium-high heat. Add the brown sugar and stir until it has somewhat dissolved.

Add the bananas and peaches to the pan and cook, stirring gently so that you don't mash up the fruit, for 3 or 4 minutes, until the fruit is glazed and the sauce is bubbly.

Pour in the rum, stir and heat until it almost simmers. Remove from the heat.

Now the fun begins. Put on a pair of oven mitts. Using a long fireplace match or barbecue-lighter, light the sauce on fire. It should flame very impressively for a couple of minutes. Make sure everyone sees this. When the flame dies out, spoon over slices of cake or regular or non-dairy ice cream. Or both. How great is that?

Makes 4 servings.

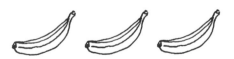

Truly Astonishing Tofu Chocolate Mousse

No really — this is amazing. It has to be tried to be believed. Not weird at all.

1 (19 oz.)	**1 (539 g)**	package silken tofu
2 cups	**500 mL**	semisweet chocolate chips

Dump the tofu into the container of a food processor or blender and blend until smooth, scraping down the sides once or twice.

Melt the chocolate chips in a small saucepan set into another saucepan filled with boiling water (or in a double boiler), stirring until smooth.

Pour the melted chocolate into the blender or processor and blend until the mixture is very smooth and creamy.

Spoon into individual dessert dishes and chill. Serve plain or with a dollop of whipped cream.

Makes about 6 very surprising servings.

Extra Added Attraction!

Use this mousse to fill a baked pie shell (or a graham cracker crust) for an amazing, decadent chocolate mousse pie. Top it, if you want, with non-dairy whipped topping or real whipped cream and sprinkle with shaved chocolate.

Rebecca's Mexican Hot Hot Chocolate

Who doesn't love a nice mug of hot chocolate on a chilly winter day? Here's one that may just knock your socks off — it's hot in more ways than one.

3 tbsp.	**45 mL**	unsweetened cocoa powder
3 tbsp.	**45 mL**	sugar
1 tsp.	**5 mL**	cinnamon
½ tsp.	**2 mL**	nutmeg
¼ tsp.	**1 mL**	cayenne pepper, or to taste (optional but amazing)
3 cups	**750 mL**	milk, regular or non-dairy, divided

In a small bowl, mix together the cocoa powder, sugar, cinnamon, nutmeg and cayenne. Pour about ¼ cup (60 mL) of the milk into the cocoa mixture and stir until smooth, without lumps. Set aside.

Pour the remaining milk into a small saucepan and place over medium-low heat. When the milk is steaming, add the cocoa mixture into the hot milk in the saucepan. Reduce the heat to low and cook for about 2 minutes, stirring constantly.

Remove from the heat and serve in your favorite mug.

Drink in front of the TV. Or the fireplace. Or wherever.

Makes about 4 servings.

Full Meal Ideas

An Evening in Athens
Authentic Greek Salad (see page 65)
Vegetarian Moussaka (see page 136)
Buttered new potatoes tossed with parsley

A Chic, but Not Obnoxious, Dinner
A whole steamed artichoke (see page 30)
Pseudo-Hollandaise Sauce (see page 30)
Roasted Tomato Sauce with fettuccine (see page 97)
Crusty French bread
Truly Astonishing Tofu Chocolate Mousse (see page 209)

A Passage to India Dinner
Potato and Green Pea Curry (see page 124)
Lentil Dal (see page 126)
Cumin-Scented Yellow Rice (see page 170)
Tomato and Cucumber Raita (see page 125)

Pan-Asian Adventure
Basic Vegetable Stir-Fry (see page 113)
Spicy Garlic Tofu and Eggplant (see page 115)
Thai Mango Salad (see page 69)
White Rice (see page 162)

A Hearty Fall Feast
Split Pea Soup (see page 40)
Zucchini and Basil Strata (see page 89)
Crunchy Carrot Salad (see page 73)
Fruit Compote (see page 207)

Flash in the Pan Dinner
Phenomenal Minestrone Soup (see page 47)
Parmesan Onion Bread (see page 196)
Peach and Banana Flambé (see page 208)

Dinner for a Dark and Stormy Night

Mushroom Barley Soup (see page 46)
Oven-Roasted Carrot and Sweet Potato Casserole (see page 140)
Bulgur Pilaf (see page 170)

A Simple but Elegant Meal

Warm Mushroom Salad with Goat Cheese (see page 62)
Easy Risotto with Asparagus (see page 169)
Fantastic Fruit Sorbet (see page 206)

A Buncha Slobs for Supper

Chock Full of Veggies Chili (see page 120)
Jalapeño Corn Bread (see page 193)
A big green salad with Creamy Greek Dressing (see page 79)
Fruit Crumble (see page 204)

When in Rome Dinner

Pasta Fagioli (see page 52)
Fabulous Focaccia (see page 192)
A mixed green salad with Balsamic Garlic Dressing (see page 78)

Summertime Blues Dinner

Basic Crepes (see page 92) filled with Ratatouille (see page 180) and
    cheese
Grilled Marinated Portobello Mushrooms (see page 153)
Corn and Tomato Salad (see page 61)
Multigrain Pilaf (see page 171)

Midnight in Moscow Dinner

Eggplant Caviar (see page 26) with dark rye bread
Old-Fashioned Potato Soup (see page 44)
Tomato-Garlic Green Beans (see page 183)
Sweet and Sour Roasted Beet Salad (see page 59)
Kasha mixed with bow-tie pasta (see page 165)

index